Surgery for Hyperopia
and Presbyopia

Surgery for Hyperopia and Presbyopia

Neal A. Sher, MD, FACS

Clinical Associate Professor of Ophthalmology
University of Minnesota Medical School

Attending Surgeon, Phillips Eye Institute
Attending Surgeon, Hennepin County Medical Center Department of Ophthalmology, and
Minneapolis Children's Medical Center

Minneapolis, Minnesota

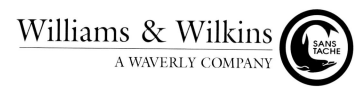

Williams & Wilkins
A WAVERLY COMPANY

BALTIMORE • PHILADELPHIA • LONDON • PARIS • BANGKOK
BUENOS AIRES • HONG KONG • MUNICH • SYDNEY • TOKYO • WROCLAW

Editor: Darlene Barela Cooke
Managing Editor: Frances M. Klass
Production Coordinator: Dana M. Soares
Typesetter: Better Graphics, Inc.
Printer: Quebecor Printing Book Group

Copyright © 1997 Williams & Wilkins

351 West Camden Street
Baltimore, Maryland 21201–2436 USA

Rose Tree Corporate Center
1400 North Providence Road
Building II, Suite 5025
Media, Pennsylvania 19063–2043 USA

Accurate indications, adverse reactions and dosage schedules for drugs are provided in this book, but it is possible that they may change. The reader is urged to review the package information data of the manufacturers of the medications mentioned.

Printed in the United States of America

First Edition,

Library of Congress Cataloging-in-Publication Data
Surgery for hyperopia and presbyopia / [edited by] Neal A. Sher,
    p.   cm.
  Includes bibliographical references and index.
  ISBN: 30333-3
  1. Presbyopia—Surgery. 2. Hyperopia—Surgery. I. Sher, Neal A.
  [DNLM: 1. Hyperopia—surgery. 2. Presbyopia—surgery. 3. Laser
Surgery.   WW 300 S961 1997]
RE938.5.S87 1997
617.7'55—dc21
DNLM/DLC   96-24160
for Library of Congress   CIP

The publishers have made every effort to trace the copyright holders for borrowed material. If they have inadvertently overlooked any, they will be pleased to make the necessary arrangements at the first opportunity.

To purchase additional copies of this book, call our customer service department at **(800) 638-0672** or fax orders to **(800) 447-8438**. For other book services, including chapter reprints and large quantity sales, ask for the Special Sales department.

Canadian customers should call **(800) 665-1148**, or fax **(800) 665-0103**. For all other calls originating outside of the United States, please call **(410) 528-4223** or fax us at **(410) 528-8550**.

Visit Williams & Wilkins on the Internet: **http://www.wwilkins.com** or contact our customer service department at **custserv@wwilkins.com**. Williams & Wilkins customer service representatives are available from 8:30 am to 6:00 pm, EST, Monday through Friday, for telephone access.

97 98 99 00
1 2 3 4 5 6 7 8 9 10

Dedication

To My Wife Judith
and Our Daughters Melissa and Cindy
Your Love and Support
Make All Endeavors Worthwhile

Foreword

It is a great pleasure and an honor to have the opportunity to write a Foreword to the groundbreaking book edited by Neal A. Sher, M.D., F.A.C.S., *Surgery for Hyperopia and Presbyopia*. Dr. Sher, along with several other distinguished individuals, enjoys a reputation as one of the world's outstanding refractive surgeons and a leading pioneer in excimer laser correction of refractive errors of the eye.

The first two chapters of this book present background information concerning the etiology and epidemiology of hyperopia and presbyopia and discuss the historical aspects of refractive surgery as it has been applied to the correction of these disorders. Subsequent chapters deal with incisional and suture techniques followed by surface photoablation and LASIK utilizing the excimer laser and other photoablative lasers as constructed by various manufacturers.

The next section deals with the various intrastromal procedures, both non-corneal contact and corneal contact, that are now being used for the correction of hyperopia. Another section discusses the latest approaches and techniques regarding the use of pseudophakic intraocular lenses and phakic intraocular lenses for the correction process. One chapter in this group deals with intracorneal lenses, and the final chapter is concerned with a new corneal contour technique and its application to the correction of hyperopia and presbyopia.

This fine work, for which Dr. Sher should be congratulated, displays a comprehensive yet incisive view of the state of the art in surgical correction of hyperopia and presbyopia. Dr. Sher brings together the finest clinical research scientists and ophthalmic intellects from around the world, who have described their various ideas and surgical approaches and techniques. The content of each of the chapters is comprehensive in nature and represents the most current thinking of the many contributors involved. This is the first refractive surgery textbook devoted entirely to the correction of hyperopia and presbyopia that combines information regarding the most recent statistics and surgical trends and eloquently positions it as the foremost treatise of its kind.

Francis A. L'Esperance Jr., M.D., F.A.C.S.
Professor of Clinical Ophthalmology
Columbia University College of Physicians and Surgeons
New York, N.Y.
USA

Preface

Someone once conjectured that the treatment of hyperopia and presbyopia is the "next frontier" of refractive surgery. This would imply that the surgical treatment of myopia is a settled issue that does not require further investigation. Although one century has past since Lans demonstrated that the cornea can be reshaped by incisions or thermal means, there is still no general agreement on the best surgical procedure for a given amount of myopia or astigmatism. The current debate concerning photorefractive keratectomy versus LASIK is just one example. Despite several safe and effective refractive procedures such as radial keratotomy and PRK, refractive surgery is a relatively new field undergoing very rapid change.

Until recently the surgical correction of hyperopia and presbyopia has lagged behind the surgery of myopia in terms of investigative efforts. The number of papers published on hyperopia have always been a small fraction of those published on myopia. There are a number of reasons for this. A cynic might conclude that research efforts have concentrated on myopia as most investigators who have a refractive error are myopic and the amount of myopa is directly correlated with intelligence. Does this mean that the smartest nearsighted investigators have been unleashed on this problem? The real answer is a combination of physiology, demographics, and economics. It is easier to permanently flatten the cornea for myopia than to steepen it centrally for hyperopia. Radial keratotomy works well to flatten the central cornea. Incisional procedures for corneal steepening such as hexagonal keratotomy are problematic at best. The preoperative uncorrected vision plays a significant role in the motivation to undergo refractive surgery; a thirty year old with myopia is more likely to seek corrective surgery than a 30 year old three diopter hyperopic individual.

Despite the above trends, I predict that there will be a rapid growth of surgery for hyperopia and presbyopia. Although refractive surgical procedures have been attempted for over 200 years, it has only been in the last 15 years that the rapid development of new technologies and entrepreneurial drive, combined with expanded patient awareness have led to a rapid growth of refractive surgery.

According to the demographics, especially in industrialized economies, many millions of "baby boomers" are now entering their late 40s and early fifties. The incidence of hyperopia (greater than 0.5 D) in this population has been estimated to be 22% in patients in their 40s increasing to almost 67% by age 65 and beyond. The incidence of presbyopia is almost universal. This group will be a prime consumer of refractive surgery, and will provide an impetus to develop safe and effective refractive surgical procedures to reduce visual handicaps.

As in myopia, there are a wide variety of surgical procedures that have been proposed for hyperopia and several other procedures for presbyopia. At present, there is little agreement on which procedure is the best for myopia and there is no consensus on hyperopic procedures. I have tried to include research being done on all aspects of this problem, including some of the most recent work, which is very preliminary.

It is a very exciting time to be an ophthalmic surgeon. Advances in ophthalmology, particularly in refractive surgery come from all over the world. The restrictive regulatory environment in the USA has tied the hands of many investigators in this country. In many cases, the leading edge technologies are now being developed and practiced in numerous places worldwide. These pioneering surgeons in Canada, South America, Europe, Australia and Asia have been generous in sharing their knowledge with their colleagues. It is an honor to be able to edit this textbook consisting of the contributions of my colleagues, many of whom I consider friends. These authors shared their insights, perspectives, experiences, both good and bad, in an effort to advance this rapidly changing field for the benefit of our patients. I am indebted to them for the huge amount of hard work and effort which goes into the preparation of each chapter.

I am indebted to the encouragement, support and friendship of Francis L'Esperance Jr., MD. His vision and genius has made the use of lasers in ophthalmology an everyday occurrence, to the benefit of millions of patients facing blindness worldwide. It was in 1965, that L'Esperance, building on the prior work of Meyer-Schwickerath, Maiman and Zweng developed systems for photocoagulation of ophthalmic vascular disease. In the 1980s, not limiting his perspective to the retina, L'Esperance saw the potential of Srinivasan and Trokel's pioneering work with ultraviolet lasers and postulated a method for corneal sculpting. This led to the formation of Taunton Technologies which later became VISX. I had the opportunity to do early excimer clinical trials with the Taunton and VISX team and had the privilege of meeting and working with Fran.

I am also grateful to Richard Lindstrom MD, a gifted surgeon, honest researcher and generous teacher for encouraging me to see the potential of refractive surgery and for his continued help and advice. I wish to thank my friends and partners in my practice, Eye Care Associates in Minneapolis including Irving Shapiro MD, the founder and guiding light of the Phillips Eye Institute, Robert Warshawsky MD, Mark Norman III, MD and Marian Rubenfeld, MD, Ph.D. They have always been supportive in my research, in giving clinical advice and in putting this book together. I appreciate the support of Bill Kelley and Eckhard Schroeder Ph.D of Aesculap-Meditec in Germany. The Meditec excimer team with their German clinical investigators was the first to demonstrate that PRK was capable of steepening the cornea and reducing hyeropia.

I also appreciate the help of Sally Zesbaugh, Janet DeMarchi, Nancy Read, Sheryl Joos and Jon Menke of Minneapolis for their assistance. A special thanks to Beth Kaufman Barry for her guidance in getting the book together and the professional editorial and production staff at Williams and Wilkins in Philadelphia and Baltimore.

Neal A. Sher, MD, FACS
Minneapolis, Minnesota, 1997

Contributors

Till Anschutz, MD
Department of Ophthalmology
Stadtklinik Baden-Baden
Laserinstitut
Baden Baden, Germany

Michael Berry, PhD
Sunrise Technologies Inc.
Fremont, California

Mark Bullimore, PhD
Ohio State University College of Optometry
Columbus, Ohio

Dieter Dausch, MD
Professor of Ophthalmology
Marienhospital Amberg
Amberg, Germany

Klaus Ditzen, MD
Eye Surgery Center Weinheim
Weinheim, Germany

Sally Donaldson, OD
Broadway Eye Surgery Center
Vancouver, Canada

Richard A. Eiferman, MD, FACS
Clinical Professor of Ophthalmology
University of Louisville
Research Service
VA Medical Center
Louisville, KY

Brad Fundingsland, BA
The Buzard Eye Institute
Las Vegas, Nevada

Bernard Gilmartin, FCOptom, PhD
Department of Vision Science
Aston University
Aston Triangle
Birmingham, United Kingdom

R. Bruce Grene, MD
CEO, Grene Vision Group
Assistant Clinical Professor, University of Kansas
    Medical Center
Witchita, Kansas

Helda Huschka, MD
Eye Surgery Center Weinheim
Weinheim, Germany

David R. Hardten, MD
Lindstrom, Samuelson & Hardten
Attending Surgeon, Phillips Eye Institute
Clinical Assistant Professor of Ophthalmology
Department of Ophthalmology, University
    of Minnesota
Director, Refractive Surgery, Department
    of Ophthalmology, St. Paul-Ramsey
    Medical Center
Minneapolis, Minnesota

Amir H.K. Isfahani, MD
Department of Ophthalmology
University of Southern California
    School of Medicine
Doheny Eye Institute
Los Angeles, California

W. Bruce Jackson, MD
Professor and Chairman
Department of Ophthalmology
University of Ottawa School of Medicine
Ottawa, Canada

Robert Klein, MD
Department of Ophthalmology
Hopital de l'Orangerie
Strasbourg, France

Douglas Koch, MD
Professor of Ophthalmology
Baylor College of Medicine
Cullen Eye Institute
Houston, Texas

Thomas Kohnen, MD
Cullen Eye Institute
Baylor College of Medicine
Houston, Texas

Colman Kraff, MD
Kraff Eye Institute
Clinical Instructor, Dept. of Ophthalmology,
    Northwestern University Medical School
Chicago, Illinois

**Michael Lawless, MBBS, MD, FRACO,
    FRACS, FRCOphth.**
Director, Sydney Refractive Surgery Center
Chief of Ophthalmology, Mater Misericordiae
    Hospital
Visiting Medical Officer in Ophthalmology,
    Royal North Shore Hospital
Royal North Shore Hospital
St. Leonards, Australia

Frances L'Esperance Jr., MD
Professor of Clinical Ophthalmology
Columbia University College of Physicians
    and Surgeons
New York, New York

Richard L. Lindstrom, MD
Clinical Professor of Ophthalmology
University of Minnesota School of Medicine
Medical Director, Center for Teaching
    and Research
Phillips Eye Institute
Minneapolis, Minnesota

Jeffrey J. Machat, MD
National Medical Co-Director
TLC The Laser Center
Toronto, Canada

Peter J. McDonnell, MD
Professor of Ophthalmology
Doheny Eye Institute
University of Southern California
Los Angeles, California

Antonio Mendez G., MD
Mendez Eye Clinic
Mexicali, Mexico

Antonio Méndez Noble, MD
Mendez Eye Clinic
Tijuana, Mexico

Richard Menefee, AAS
Sunrise Technologies Inc.
Fremont, CA

Robert Nordquist, PhD
Wound Healing of Oklahoma, Inc
Oklahoma City, OK

Marc G. Odrich, MD
Assistant Professor of Clinical Ophthalmology
Columbia University College of Physicians
    and Surgeons
New York, New York

Louis Probst, MD
Assistant Professor, Cornea and
    Refractive Surgery
University of Western Ontario
London, Canada
Medical Director
TLC The Windsor Laser Center
Windsor, Canada

James Salz, MD
Clinical Professor of Ophthalmology
University of Southern California
Los Angeles, California

Daljit Singh, MD
Amristar, India

Peter Stockdill, MD, FRCS(C)
Clinical Assistant Professor, Dept. of
    Ophthalmology, University of British Columbia
Consultant, Langley Memorial Hospital
Langley, British Columbia

Hugo Sutton, MD
Broadway Eye Surgery Centre
Vancouver, Canada

Casimir Swinger, MD
Professor of Ophthalmology
Mt. Sinai School of Medicine
New York, New York

Vance Thompson, MD
Clinical Assistant Professor, University of South
    Dakota Medical School
Director of Refractive Surgery, Sioux Valley
    Memorial Hospital
Sioux Valley, South Dakota

Spencer Thornton, MD, FACS
Director of Clinical Research, and Medical
    Director, Thornton Eye Center
Nashville, Tennessee

Rogelio V. Villarreal, MD
Doheny Eye Institute
University of Southern California
Los Angeles, California

Paolo Vinciguerra, MD
Department of Ophthalmology
Saint Gerardo Hospital
Monza, Italy

Contents

section I
Background

CHAPTER 1

Hyperopia and Presbyopia: Etiology and Epidemiology

Mark A. Bullimore
Bernard Gilmartin

INTRODUCTION

Hyperopia and presbyopia are unavoidably linked and confused in the minds of the lay public because they elucidate identical symptoms, namely difficulty with near vision. Although the ramifications of these two conditions are very similar, the prevalence and etiology are dramatically different. Hyperopia affects a relatively small proportion of the population. Conversely, presbyopia can be viewed in the same way as death and taxes; inevitable. Hyperopia is caused by a mismatch in the refractive and axial components of the eye. On the other hand, presbyopia is a result of a failure of the accommodative mechanism, although the precise etiology remains the subject of some debate. This chapter reviews the etiology and epidemiology of hyperopia and presbyopia, although as will become apparent, large gaps exist in the literature.

THE ETIOLOGY AND PREVALENCE OF HYPEROPIA

Hyperopia occurs when the refracting optics of the eye are to weak relative to the length of the eye, with images of distant objects being brought to focus behind the retina (Fig. 1–1). This occurs either when the cornea and lens power are too weak in an eye of normal size, or when the cornea and lens power are normal but the eye is too short.

Although there is a wealth of literature and energetic debate about the etiology of myopia,[1] hyperopia has been pretty well ignored.[2] This imbalance in the scientific literature is likely due to a number of factors. First myopia is progressive, whereas hyperopia is relatively stable. Second, severe myopia has a number of unpleasant sequelae, such

as retinal detachment, from which the hyperopia eye is relatively immune. Finally myopia is more prevalent, particularly among the intelligent individuals who might be inclined to study refractive errors.

Most studies of infant refractive error conclude that newborns are moderately hyperopic but have a broad distribution of refractive errors (Fig. 1–2). Between infancy and childhood two things occur. First, the eye grows in such a way that the mean refractive error shifts towards emmetropia, second the distribution narrows considerably. These trends combine to produce a steady reduction in the prevalence of hyperopia. It is then perhaps curious that Hirsch[3] found a prevalence of around 25% in 13–14 year olds. There are also some reports that hyperopia increases between the ages of 3 and 7 years[4–6] but it is very likely that these data arise from sampling artifacts.

In contrast to myopia that progresses steadily, hyperopia tends to persist throughout childhood. As mentioned above, most infants begin life with a moderate degree of hyperopia. The process of emmetropization[7] then results in a reduction in the amount and the frequency of hyperopia (Table 1–1), as well as a narrowing of the distribution of refractive error (Fig. 1–2). Hyperopia could thus represent a failure of the emmetropization mechanism or an initial level of hyperopia so extreme that emmetropization could not overcome it. Recent longitudinal evidence suggests that the former is true. In a study of 93 infants with at least +4.00 D of hyperopia at age 9 months, the average change by age 3.5 years was a decrease in hyperopia, but only by −0.50 to −0.75 D.[11] In a study of 65 infants refracted during the first six months of life and again between ages 9 and 16 years, 18 of 20 children with some degree of hyperopia in infancy were nonmyopic in childhood.[12]

A

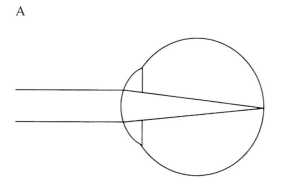

B

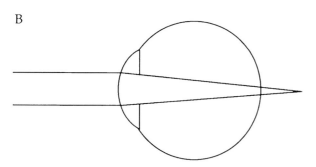

Fig. 1–1. Schematic representations of A the emmetropic eye and B the hyperopic eye.

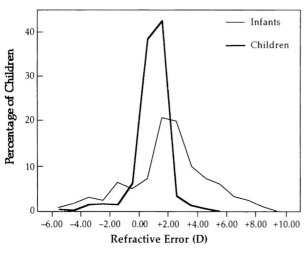

Fig. 1–2. Distribution of refractive errors in newborn
infants (Cook and Glasscock[10]) and children (Mutti and
Zadnik[14]). Note that the distribution for children is nar-
rower. Redrawn from Mutti and Zadnik.[14]

Slow ocular growth may both be the reason for
the appearance of hyperopia as well as why it does
not disappear with time. Hyperopia refractions are
associated with shorter axial lengths, shallower
anterior chamber depths, and flatter corneas.[13]
Previous literature suggests that lens power is not
correlated with hyperopia, but recent work suggests
correlations of ~0.2, with hyperopes having
steeper, more powerful lenses than other subjects.[14]
In summary much is still to be learned about the
developing eye, particularly with respect to hyperopia.

Hyperopia in Adulthood

Refractive error is relatively stable in adulthood.
Slataper[6] showed an increase in average myopia up
to age 20 years in a large clinical sample consisting
of cycloplegic refractions in over thirty thousand
eyes (Fig. 1–3). This is consistent with the notion
that eye growth and the progression of myopia are
largely complete by adulthood. Little change is seen
up to the age of 50 years, at which point, there
begins a marked increase in hyperopia. Wang et
al.[15] recently reported the prevalence of refractive
errors in 4926 adults over 43 years of age (Table
1–2). They found that hyperopia is much more common at age 65–74 years (67%) than it is at age
43–54 years (22%).

The underlying cause of this hyperopic shift is still
unknown. It is well known that the crystalline lens
both thickens and steepens during this time[16] but
this implies that eyes should become more *myopic*
with age, leading to a phenomenon often referred to
as "the lens paradox." Grosvenor has suggested that
the length of the eye actually shrinks with age in
order to prevent this myopia.[17] Recent studies propose that the gradient refractive index structure of
the lens changes so that the net equivalent index
of the lens decreases, and so does its equivalent
power.[18] In summary, the lens radii of curvature
may steepen, but this refractive index change causes
a net shift toward hyperopia.

The paucity of literature on hyperopia extends to
its epidemiology and little has been published on
risk factors or associations. Of interest is the recent
finding that hyperopia is significantly correlated
(r = −0.32) with education level, less educated individuals having more hyperopia.[15] The same data
set failed to show a relationship between an associ-

Table 1–1. Prevalence of Hyperoia in Children

Author(s)	N	Critrion	Method	Age (years)	Prevalence
Kempf et al.[4]		>+1.00 D	Cycloplegic retinoscopy	6–8	35.4%
				9–11	25.2%
				12 and above	15.2%
Blum et al.[8]	>1,000	≥+1.50 D	Noncycloplegic retinoscopy	5–15	6%
Hirsch[3]	261	>+1.00 D	Noncycloplegic retinoscopy	13–14	26.4%
Laatikainen and Erkkila[9]	162	≥+2.00 D	Cycloplegic retinoscopy	7–8	19.1%
	218			9–10	6.9%
	222			11–12	11.7%
	220			14–15	3.6%

ation between refractive error and either household income or occupation.

THE ETIOLOGY OF PRESBYOPIA

Our understanding of the etiology of presbyopia is derived principally from our understanding of the mechanism of accommodation in young eyes. Helmholtz did much to clarify these mechanisms[19] but despite much research in the last hundred years there is still no consensus on the precise mechanism of accommodation due, in part, to the lack of an easily accessible animal model.

The Mechanism of Accommodation in Young Eyes

The accommodative apparatus is driven principally by parasympathetic innervation of the ciliary smooth muscle. This causes the muscle to slide forward in a unified manner and produce an inward movement of the muscle. The result is a reduction in the diameter of the ciliary muscle collar that instigates a series of events leading to an ability to see near objects clearly: relaxation of tension of the zonular fibers; release of inherent viscoelastic properties of the lens capsule and lens substance; axial thickening of the nucleus of the lens; decrease in anterior lens radius; central bulging of the anterior central region of the lens; increase in dioptric power of the lens.

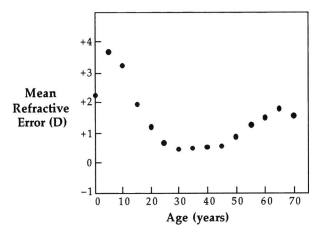

Fig. 1–3. Average refractive error as a function of age (after Slataper[6]).

Table 1–2. Prevalence of Hyperopia (>+0.50 D) in Adults[15]

Age Range (years)	N	Prevalence
43–54	1,468	22.1%
55–64	1,232	50.2%
65–74	1,089	67.2%
75+	486	68.5%

Magnetic resonance imaging (MRI) of the eye can now be used for *in vivo* study of the dynamics of accommodation due to the improved resolution afforded by special coil attachments[20] but early illustrations of the above processes were provided by Brown's Scheimpflug photographs[21-23]. Brown's series of photographs were used to demonstrate changes in cross-sectional lens dimensions induced by accommodative stimuli of up to −10 D. The photographs clearly demonstrate that the amplitude of accommodation decreases with age and that the zones of discontinuity of the lens merge in the older eyes. Lack of mobility was also seen to be associated with thickening of the lens together with a decrease in anterior radii of curvature to a level not found for normal accommodation responses in young eyes.

Changes in Crystalline Lens Dimensions with Age

The changes in lens dimensions with age are substantial, including a 33% increase in volume between 30 and 60 years of age. These are likely to be a major factor in the etiology of presbyopia. Brown found an average increase in lens thickness of around 1 mm,[21] a finding confirmed with ultrasound measurement in more recent studies,[24] which was attributed mainly to the lens cortex; the dimensions of the lens nucleus appear to remain constant throughout life. A consequence of these relationships is a gradual decrease in anterior radius of the lens with age of, on average, around 5 mm between 20 and 60 years-of-age.

The Geometry of Zonular Attachments

Compensation for the increase in size of the lens appears to also take place in relation to the zonular attachments. Farnsworth and her colleagues reported on changes in zonular insertion with age and hypothesized that the associated change in geometry of the attachments might be a factor in the development of presbyopia.[25,26] Photographs of the anterior crystalline lens surfaces of 17-, 46- and 85-year old individuals were used to illustrate the relative migration forward of the zonular attachments across the face of the lens as the lens diameter increased with age. The migrations could be interpreted as a consequence of the apparent constancy of zonule dimensions and elasticity over an

individual's life but their role in the development of presbyopia is equivocal as the most significant shifts in attachment sites were found to occur after the onset of presbyopia.

Some years later Koretz and her associates presented systematic analyses of the biophysics and mathematics of the changing geometrical relationships between zonule and lens as lens size increased with age.[27-30] The principal observation was that with increased lens size the zonular insertions would become more tangential to the lens surface and thus would be less able to impart tension on the lens capsule. By comparing data pertaining to accommodating, nonaccommodating and presbyopic eyes the approach has allowed progress to be made in simulation of the effect of age on the facility that the lens matrix has to modify its internal configuration. An important prerequisite for the model adopted by these workers was to specify that the lens capsule acts as a uniform 'force distributor,' that is, the tractions exerted by the zonular apparatus on the capsule are spread evenly over the lens fiber surface. Subsequent work on microfluctuations of accommodation has provided some support for this view[31] although the idea conflicts with early work that proposed that it is variations in thickness of the lens capsule that determine the configuration of the lens matrix during accommodation.[32] Recent work on lens capsule dimensions provides support for this proposal.[33]

Viscoelastic Properties of the Lens

Whatever stance is taken on the topography of forces imposed by the capsule it is clear that capsular elasticity diminishes with age. *In vitro* data on the viscoelastic properties of lens capsule and lens matrix collected by Fisher indicates clearly that the ability of the capsule to mold the lens wanes as we get older. Young's modulus of capsular elasticity is reduced by a factor of two by the mid-40s.[34,35] In the young eye the modulus of elasticity of the lens matrix is several orders of magnitude less than the capsule and it is thus compliant with the molding pressure of the capsule. Fisher has shown, however, that the efficacy of this response also diminishes with age. When taking the difference in molding pressure between polar and equatorial regions of the lens as an index of the facility for central anterior bulging of the lens, it was shown that the difference *increases* by a factor of around two by the mid-40's.[36–38] Hence the inexorable decline in near focusing ability with age is associated with a decline in the ability of the viscoelastic system to both apply molding pressure and to respond to the molding pressure.

Extralenticular Causes of Presbyopia

Although there is compelling evidence that presbyopia results principally from age-related dysfunction of the crystalline lens it should be emphasized that there is no evidence for sclerosis of the lens with age.[39,40] Interest in recent years in the contribution of extralenticular structures to the process of accommodation has led to consideration of their relevance to presbyopia.[41–44]

A relatively straightforward explanation of presbyopia would follow if it could be shown that the ciliary muscle lost its ability to contract with age. Unfortunately there is no evidence that this occurs; in fact Fisher has shown using postmortem material that the contractile force of the ciliary muscle reaches a maximum at around 45 years-of-age.[45] Later work on monkeys used standard histological criteria to show that the ciliary muscle of very old animals is capable of contracting enough to produce substantial levels of accommodation.[46–48] Of importance, however, is not force of the muscle contraction but rather the movement of the muscle: it is the movement that produces the change in geometric configuration of the ciliary muscle and subsequently the reduction in diameter of the ciliary collar that is necessary for accommodation to occur.

Ciliary muscle contraction without inward muscle movement has been demonstrated (at least in qualitative terms) in a series of experiments on monkeys using Scheimpflug- and gonio-videography of the anterior segment.[49] The ciliary processes were used as reference points to observe *in vivo* the inward centripetal movement of the ciliary body (and hence muscle) on electrical stimulation of the Edinger-Westphal nucleus via an implanted electrode. For young monkeys an inwards excursion of the ciliary processes could be clearly seen in the video pictures. For older monkeys there was a virtual absence of any excursion even though the ciliary muscle was receiving and able to respond to maximum stimulation. There was thus no opportunity for the older eye to generate genuine accommoda-

tion because immobilization of inward movement of the ciliary muscle did not permit release of zonular tension. The findings have attracted attention and have prompted renewed examination of the biomechanical aspects of the component elements of the accommodative process.[50–52]

Biomechanics of Ciliary Muscle Contraction

The ciliary muscle is attached anteriorly by means of tendons to the scleral spur and trabecular meshwork and posteriorly to the elastic network of Bruch's membrane of the choroid. The posterior attachment is in turn linked to the scleral canal and hence to postequatorial sections of the globe. It is clear that posteriorly there needs to be a firm point of attachment and this is provided by anchoring ligaments in the pars plana region that provide an inherent restraining elastic force for the posterior zonular fiber system. The anterior fiber system (the zonular plexus which divides to attach to anterior and posterior parts of the lens capsule) is linked to the posterior system by an intermediate tensile fiber system. These intermediate fibers attach firmly to the ciliary crypts and whilst their function is not fully understood they represent an important biomechanical fulcrum that provides the fine leverage necessary for fast and precise changes in accommodations.[53–57]

Thus in an unaccommodated state the elasticity of the anchoring ligaments produces a decrease in tension in the tensile fiber system but a concomitant increase in tension in the anterior zonules, which leads to lens flattening. On contraction of the ciliary muscle the forward and inward movement of the muscle causes stretching of the tension fiber system such that traction is taken up from the posterior zonular fibers (and the choroid) that allows relaxation of the anterior zonules and subsequent lens thickening. The accommodation following ciliary muscle contraction could thus be considered as a process whereby energy is stored in the posterior fiber system for subsequent release when innervation of the ciliary muscle ceases. The corollary is, therefore, that in the young eye the anchor region is continually applying an anterior-posterior force that maintains the eye in a unaccommodated or disaccommodated state. The forward movement of the ciliary muscle on contraction counters the stretch in this system and allows relaxation of the zonular fibers and subsequent thickening of the crystal-line lens. We can thus envisage accommodation as a neuromuscular process that modulates (in the young eye) an inherent bias towards an unaccommodated state.[58]

Dysfunction of Posterior Attachments of the Ciliary Muscle

The above account of the biomechanics of accommodation has led to proposals that in the presbyopic eye dysfunction of the peripheral anchors prevents ciliary muscle contraction (however strong) from inducing the necessary inward movement of the muscle and so account for the lack of ciliary muscle movement found in the nerve stimulation work on monkeys cited earlier.[49,58]

One proposal is that the posterior elastic anchor tissue becomes flaccid and thus allows the ciliary muscle to move forward and inward so that the lens will assume an accommodated state;[59] there is some evidence that this occurs with age at least for the lens cortex.[22] Once this has occurred, innervation of the ciliary muscle will only be able to cause contraction of the muscle and not the inward movement necessary for accommodation.

A separate proposal is of particular interest as it has received support from histochemical and ultra-structural studies of connective tissue at the posterior aspect of the ciliary muscle.[60,61] Rather than becoming flaccid it is suggested that with the onset of presbyopia the posterior elastic anchor tissues become rigid, the result being that ciliary muscle contraction can occur but is again unable to produce the necessary inward movement for accommodation.

THE EPIDEMIOLOGY OF PRESBYOPIA

As pointed out by Kleinstein,[62] presbyopia is a chronic condition with a "slow, indefinite onset." Its prevalence can be considered to be 100% by the age of 50 years if the eye's depth of focus is taken into account.[63] Age of onset of presbyopia does not appear to vary with gender, although, intuitively, individuals of lesser stature would be expected to experience symptoms at an earlier age by virtue of their shorter arms. Earlier onset of presbyopia may also be precipitated in systemic diseases such

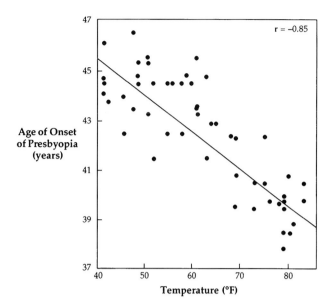

Fig. 1–4. The relationship between age of onset of presbyopia and temperature in 53 cities (after Miranda[66]).

as diabetes or myasthenia gravis, by prescription and nonprescription drugs,[64] and following ocular trauma.

One aspect that has received some attention is that of geographic location.[65] Although race does not appear to systematically affect the age of onset of presbyopia, the ambient temperature of the environment seems to have a significant affect.[65] Miranda[66] showed that presbyopia occurs earlier in countries closer to the equator (Fig. 1–4).

SUMMARY

We regard presbyopia, not as a disease, but as a part of the normal aging process. This perception can breed complacency about its prevention. Nonetheless, its annoying consequences and a prevalence of 100% make it an attractive subject for research by scientists and industry alike.

REFERENCES

1. Mutti DO, Zadnik K, Adams AJ: Myopia: The nature versus nurture debate goes on. *Invest Ophthalmol Vis Sci* 37:952–957, 1996.

2. Grosvenor T: The neglected hyperope. *Am J Optom Arch Am Acad Optom* 48:376–382, 1971.

3. Hirsch MJ: Predictability of refraction at age 14 on the basis of testing at age 6—interim report from the Ojai Longitudinal Study of Refraction. *Am J Optom Arch Am Acad Optom* 41:567–573, 1964.

4. Kempf GA, Collins SD, Jarman BL: Refractive errors in the eyes of children as determined by retinoscopic examination with a cycloplegic. Public Health Bulletin No. 182. USPHS, Washington, D.C., 1928.

5. Brown EVL: Net average yearly changes in refraction of atropinized eyes from birth to beyond middle life. *Arch Ophthalmol* 13:719–734, 1938.

6. Slataper FJ: Age norms of refraction and vision. *Arch Ophthalmol* 43:466–481, 1950.

7. van Alphen GWHM: On emmetropia and ametropia. *Ophthalmologica Supplementum* 142:1–92, 1961.

8. Blum HL, Peters HB, Bettman JW: *Vision Screening for Elementary Schools: The Orinda Study.* Berkeley, University of California Press, 1959.

9. Laatikainen L, Erkkila H: Visual screening of school children. *Acta Ophthalmol (Copenhagen)* 1980; 58(1): 137–143.

10. Cook RC, Glasscock RE: Refractive and ocular findings in the newborn. *Am J Ophthalmol* 34:1407–1413, 1951.

11. Atkinson J: Infant vision screening: Prediction and prevention of strabismus and amblyopia from refractive screening in the Cambridge Photorefraction Program. In K Simons: *Early Visual Development Normal and Abnormal.* New York, Oxford University Press, 1993.

12. Gwiazda J, Thorn F, Bauer J, Held R: Emmetropization and the progression of manifest refraction in children followed from infancy to puberty. *Clin Vis Sci* 8:337–344, 1993.

13. Mutti DO, Zadnik K: The utility of three predictors of childhood myopia: A Bayesian analysis. *Vision Res* 35:1345–1352, 1995.

14. Mutti DO, Zadnik K: Refractive Error. In Zadnik K: *The Optometric Examination: Measurements and Findings.* Orlando, WB Saunders, in press.

15. Wang Q, Klein BEK, Klein R, Moss SE: Refractive status in the Beaver Dam Eye Study. *Invest Ophthalmol Vis Sci* 35:4344–4347, 1994.

16. Brown N: The change in lens curvature with age. *Exp Eye Res* 19:175–183, 1974.

17. Grosvenor T: Reduction in axial length with age: An emmetropizing mechanism for the adult eye? *Am J Optom Physiol Opt* 64:657–663, 1987.

18. Hemenger RP, Garner LF, Ooi CS: Change with age of the refractive index gradient of the human ocular lens. *Invest Ophthalmol Vis Sci* 36:703–707, 1995.

19. von Helmholtz HV: Ueber die Accommodation des Auges. Graefes *Arch Ophthalmol* 1:1–74, 1855.

20. Strenk SA, Semmlow JL, Mezrich RS: Using magnetic resonance imaging to mathematically model the lens capsule. *Invest Ophthalmol Vis Sci* (Suppl) 35: 1948, 1994.

21. Brown NP: The change in shape and internal form of the lens of the eye in accommodation. *Exp Eye Res* 15:441–459, 1973.

22. Brown NP: Lens change with age and cataract; slit-image photography. In *The Human Lens in Relation to Cataract* (CIBA Symposium Foundation). Amsterdam, Netherlands, Elsevier, 1973, pp. 65–78.

23. Brown NP: The shape of the lens equator. *Exp Eye Res* 20:571–576, 1974.

24. Koretz JF, Kaufman PL, Neider MW, Goeckner PA: Accommodation and presbyopia in the human eye—aging of the anterior segment. *Vision Res* 29:1685–1692, 1989.

25. Farnsworth PN, Burke P: Three-dimensional architecture of the suspensory apparatus of the lens of the rhesus monkey. *Exp Eye Res* 25:563–577, 1977.

26. Farnsworth PN, Shyne SE: Anterior zonular shifts with age. *Exp Eye Res* 28:291–297, 1979.

27. Koretz JF, Handleman GH: Model of the accommodative mechanism in the human eye. *Vision Res* 22:917–924, 1982.

28. Koretz JF, Handelman GHA: A model for accommodation in the young human eye: The effects of lens elastic anisotropy on the mechanism. *Vision Res* 23:1679–1686, 1983.

29. Koretz JF, Handelman GH, Brown NP: Analysis of human crystalline lens curvature as a function of accommodative state and age. *Vision Res* 24:1141–1151, 1984.

30. Koretz JF, Bertasso AM, Neider WM, True-Gabelt B, Kaufman PL: Slit-lamp studies of the rhesus monkey eye. II. Changes in crystalline lens shape, thickness and position during accommodation and aging. *Exp Eye Res* 45:317–326, 1987.

31. Winn B, Pugh JR, Gilmartin B, Owens H: The frequency characteristics of accommodative microfluctuations for central and peripheral zones of the crystalline lens. *Vision Res* 30:1093–1099, 1990.

32. Fincham EF: The mechanism of accommodation. *Br J Ophthalmol Monogr Suppl VIII,* 1–80, 1937.

33. Travers MJA: Structural correlates of shape change in the primate crystalline lens. Unpublished PhD Thesis, The City University, London, UK, 1990.

34. Fisher RF: Elastic constants of the human lens capsule. *J Physiol (Lond)* 201:1–19, 1969.

35. Fisher RF: The significance of the shape of the lens and capsular energy changes in accommodation. *J Physiol (Lond)* 201:21–47, 1969.

36. Fisher RF: The elastic constants of the human lens. *J Physiol (Lond)* 212:147–180, 1971.

37. Fisher RF: Human lens fibre transparency and mechanical stress. *Exp Eye Res* 16:41–49, 1973.

38. Fisher RF: Presbyopia and the changes with age in the human crystalline lens. *J Physiol (Lond)* 228:765–779, 1973.

39. Pierscionek BK, Weale RA: Presbyopia—a maverick of human aging. *Arch Gerontol Geriatrics,* in press.

40. Fisher RF, Pettet BE: Presbyopia and the water content of the human crystalline lens. *J Physiol (Lond)* 234:443–447, 1973.

41. Crawford KS, Kaufman PL, Bito LZ: The role of the iris in accommodation of rhesus monkeys. *Invest Ophthalmol Vis Sci* 31:2185–2190, 1990.

42. Coleman DJ: On the hydraulic suspension theory of accommodation. *Trans Am Ophthalmol Soc* 84:846–868, 1986.

43. Fisher RF: The vitreous and lens in accommodation. *Trans Ophthal Soc UK* 102:318–322, 1983.

44. Schachar RA, Cudmore DP, Torti R, Black TD, Huang TA: A physical model demonstrating Schachar's hypothesis of accommodation. *Ann Ophthalmol* 26:4–9, 1994.

45. Fisher RF: The force of contraction of the human ciliary muscle during accommodation. *J Physiol (Lond)* 270:51–74, 1977.

46. Poyer JF, Kaufman PL, Flügel C: Age does not affect contractile responses of the isolated rhesus monkey ciliary muscle to muscarinic agonists. *Curr Eye Res* 12:413–422, 1993.

47. Lütjen-Drecoll E, Tamm E, Kaufman PL: Age changes in rhesus monkey ciliary muscle: Light and electron microscopy. *Exp Eye Res* 47:885–899, 1988.

48. Lütjen-Drecoll E, Tamm E, Kaufman PL: Age-related loss of morphologic responses to pilocarpine in rhesus monkey ciliary muscle. *Arch Ophthalmol* 106:1591–1598, 1988.

49. Neider MW, Crawford K, Kaufman PL, Bito LZ: In vivo videography of the rhesus monkey accommodative apparatus. *Arch Ophthalmol* 108:69–74, 1990.

50. Stark L: Presbyopia in the light of accommodation. *Am J Optom Physiol Opt* 65:407–416, 1988.

51. Wyatt JH: Application of a simple mechanical model of accommodation to the aging eye. *Vision Res* 33:731–738, 1994.

52. Beers APA,, Van Der Heijde GL: *In vivo* determination of the biomechanical properties of the component elements of the accommodation mechanism. *Vision Res* 34:2897–2905, 1994.

53. Weale RA: *The senescence of human vision.* Oxford, Oxford University Press, 1992.

54. Rohen JW, Rentsch FJ: Der Konstrucktive Bau des Zonulaaparates beim Menschem und dessen funktionelle Bedeutung. *Graefes ARch Klin Exp Ophthalmol* 178:1–19, 1969.

55. Davanger M: The suspensory apparatus of the lens. The surface of the ciliary body. A scanning electron microscopic study. *Acta Ophthalmol (Copenh)* 53:19–33, 1975.

56. Rohen JW: Scanning electron microscopic studies of the zonular apparatus in human and monkey eyes. *Invest Ophthalmol Vis Sci* 18:133–144, 1979.

57. Ober M, Rohen JW: Regional differences in the fine structure of the ciliary epithelium related to accommodation. *Invest Ophthalmol Vis Sci* 18:655–664, 1979.

58. Kaufman PL: Accommodation and presbyopia: neuromuscular and biophysical aspects. In Hart WM Jr (ed): *Adler's Physiology of the Eye, Clinical Application.* 9th ed, pp. 391–411, St Louis, Mosby, 1992.

59. Bito LZ, Miranda OC: Presbyopia, the need for a closer look. In Stark L and Obrecht G: *Presbyopia* New York, Fairchild Publications, pp. 411–429, 1987.

60. Tamm E. Lütjen-Drecoll E, Jungkunz W, Rohen JW: Posterior attachment of the ciliary muscle in young, accommodating old, presbyopic rhesus monkeys. *Invest Ophthalmol Vis Sci* 32:1678–1692, 1991.

61. Tamm E, Croft MA, Jungkunz W, Rohen JW: Age-related loss of ciliary muscle mobility in the rhesus monkey; role of the choroid. *Arch Ophthalmol* 110:871–876, 1992.

62. Kleinstein RN: Epidemiology of presbyopia. In Stark LW and Obrecht G (eds): *Presbyopia.* New York, Fairchild Publications, 1987, pp. 12–18.

63. Hamasaki D, Ong J, Marg E: The amplitude of accommodation in presbyopia. *Am J Optom Arch Am Acad Optom* 33:3–14, 1956.

64. Roy FH: *Ocular differential diagnosis.* Philadelphia, Lea and Febiger, 1984.

65. Weale RA: Human ocuar aging and ambient temperature. *Br J Ophthalmol* 65:869–870, 1981.

66. Miranda MN: The environmental factor in the onset of presbyopia. In Stark LW and Obrecht G (eds): *Presbyopia.* New York, Fairchild Publications, 1987, pp. 19–27.

CHAPTER 2

Surgery for Hyperopia: An Historical Perspective

Bradley Fundingsland
Neal A. Sher

INTRODUCTION

The surgical correction of myopia through radial keratotomy, photorefractive keratectomy and laser assisted keratomileusis (LASIK) has gained overwhelming support in the literature and among the ophthalmic community as a whole. In contrast, hyperopic refractive error has yet to find a broadly accepted means of surgical correction. Techniques conducted with fluctuating frequency over the past century include the reshaping of the cornea through incisions, burns, laser ablations, lamellar cuts and the replacement of the posterior lens.[1] This chapter will briefly review the historical development of some of these procedures.

HEXAGONAL KERATOTOMY

Hexagonal keratotomy is designed to steepen corneal curvature through the use of six corneal incisions made in a hexagonal pattern. This permits the incisions to gape open thus weakening the corneal periphery. This weakening steepens the cornea, increasing the central curvature and the overall corneal refractive power (see Fig. 2–1). This procedure has been used to correct radial keratotomy overcorrections, miscalculation of intraocular lens power and primary hyperopia.

In 1952, Akiyama[2] working with innovations developed by Sato, first described the ability of posterior hexagonal incisions to correct hyperopia in rabbits. Yamashita, in 1979, experimented with an anterior cornea incisional technique in rabbits for creating peripheral flattening and reported his results in 1986.[3] He termed this approach hexagonal keratotomy. This research, in addition to work by Gills,[4] contributed to the first presentation of

clinical data by Mendez in 1986 and the first clinical publication on hexagonal keratotomy reported by Neumann in 1988.[5] In this study, Neumann reduced hyperopia from a preoperative mean of 3.2 diopters to 1.0 diopter.

Early applications of hexagonal keratotomy[5,6] utilized a technique of six confluent, intersecting incisions in the shape of a hexagon with an optical zone of 4.5 mm to 6.0 mm as defined by Mendez[6] (Fig. 2–2). Despite the ability of the Mendez procedure to reduce hyperopia, the technique tended to isolate the central cornea leading to poor wound healing, scarring, and global rupture.[7,8] An early series by Mendez, reported by Jensen, showed the results of hexagonal keratotomy in 102 eyes, with a preoperative hyperopia ranged from +2.0 to +8.0 D. He reported an average correction of 1.50 +/− 0.75 D with a hexagon of 6.0 mm in diameter. An average correction of 2.00 +/− 0.75 D was achieved with an 5.5 mm hexagon and 3.0 +/− 0.75 D was achieved with a 5.0 mm hexagon. At that time, the corners were connected. Uncorrected visual acuity was increased to 20/20 in 36% of the eyes, 20/25 to 20/40 in 41%, and 20/50 to 20/200 in 25% of the eyes.[9]

In order to rectify this problem, Jensen[9] in 1989, introduced the use on nonintersecting hexagonal incisions. This approach increased relative safety but reduced the amount of hyperopic correction. In order to increase the range of this procedure, Mendez and Jensen further modified hexagonal techniques to increase the amount of correction by adding additional transverse incisions to the periphery that increases corneal curvature and squares up both ends of each incision. These modifications include the use of t-hex pattern in which the six incision hexagon is bounded by six transverse incisions.[10,11] (Fig. 2–3) and the use of an arcuate hex

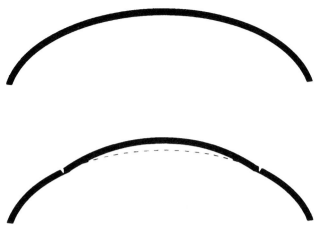

Fig. 2–1. Hexagonal keratotomy consists of six corneal incisions made in a hexagonal pattern. This permits the incisions to gape open thus weakening the corneal periphery. This weakening steepens the cornea, increasing the central curvature and the overall corneal refractive power.

incision where the six incision hexagon is followed with two arcuate incisions 6 to 8 months postoperatively.[12]

Little data has been reported on this procedure in the literature. Jensen reported the results of 483 eyes operated between 1987 and 1990 and reported a mean decrease in hyperopia of 2.25 diopter but

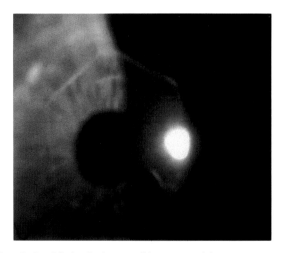

Fig. 2–2. Clinical photo of hexagonal keratotomy with 6 intersecting incisions.

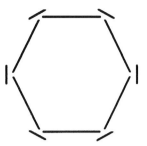

Fig. 2–3. Modified hexagonal techniques to increase the amount of correction by adding additional transverse incisions to the periphery which increases corneal curvature and squares up both ends of each incision. These modifications include the use of t-hex pattern in which the 6 incision hexagon is bounded by 6 transverse incisions.

little data was presented.[9] In 1992, Nordan and Maxwell strongly advocated avoiding hexagonal keratotomy due to the complications of irregular astigmatism and the loss of best corrected spectacle acuity (BSCVA).[13] Overall, hexagonal keratotomy has been found to lack consistent outcomes and has led to significant complications. Some of these are detailed below.

Complications of Hexagonal Keratotomy

Basuk et al.[7] reported a series of complications after hexagonal keratotomy in 15 eyes of 10 patients. These complications included glare, photophobia, polyopia, fluctuation in vision, overcorrection, irregular astigmatism, corneal edema, corneal perforation, bacterial keratitis, cataract and endophthalmitis. Wound healing abnormalities and anterior displacement of the central cornea adjacent to the incisions were common. Eight of fifteen eyes lost BSCVA of two or more Snellen lines. Three eyes required penetrating keratoplasty for visual rehabilitation.

Figure 2–4A and B shows a slit lamp photo and photokeratograph from the Basuk series of a 35 year old woman who had previously undergone radial keratotomy with 24 incisions and had hexagonal keratotomy for presbyopic symptoms. The patient had scars 80–90% of the corneal thickness and were irregularly spaced. The hexagonally arranged scars intersected the radial ones, reached

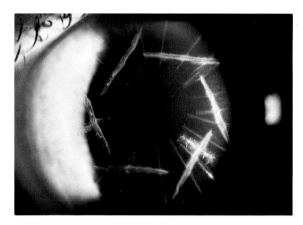

A

70 to 80% of the corneal thickness and appeared to be filled with epithelial plugs. The patient had best corrected acuity of 20/40 and intractable foreign body sensation and symptoms of visual distortion. She was fitted with a rigid gas permeable contact lens but was intolerant because of pain.

Figure 2–5 shows another case from the same series, a 45 year old woman who underwent hexagonal keratotomy and transverse keratotomy a month later. The cornea was edematous and slightly elevated. Some of the incisions gaped significantly, and contained inclusions cysts. BSCVA was 20/60.

Figure 2–6 is another example of the severe scarring that can occur after hexagonal incisions cross radial incisions.

Hexagonal keratotomy appears to have an unacceptably high complication rate that is attributable to poor wound healing and a destabilized cornea and is a procedure that should not be performed.

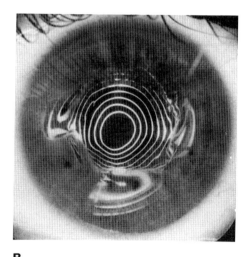

B

Fig. 2–4. *A* and *B* shows a slit lamp photo and photokeratograph from the Basuk series[7] of a 35 year old woman who had previously undergone radial keratotomy with 24 incisions and had hexagonal keratotomy for presbyopic symptoms. The patient had scars 80–90% of the corneal thickness and were irregularly spaced. The patient had best corrected acuity of 20/40 and intractable foreign body sensation and symptoms of visual distortion. She was fitted with a rigid gas permeable contact lens but was intolerant because of pain. (Printed with permission, American Journal of Ophthalmology and author.)

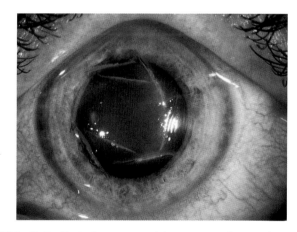

Fig. 2–5. Forty-five year old woman who underwent hexagonal keratotomy and transverse keratotomy a month later. The cornea was edematous and slightly elevated. Some of the incisions gaped significantly, and contained inclusions cysts. BSCVA was 20/60. (Printed with permission, American Journal of Ophthalmology.)

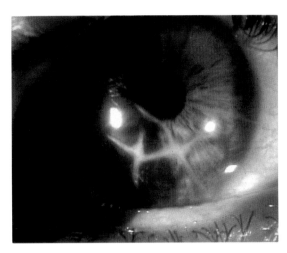

Fig. 2–6. Another example of the severe scarring which can occur after hexagonal incisions cross radial incisions. (Print in color.)

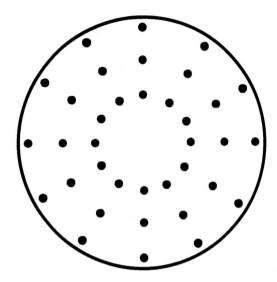

Fig. 2–7. Thermokeratoplasty involves making a series of deep burns in radially oriented spots throughout the cornea.

THERMOKERATOPLASTY

Thermokeratoplasty involves making a series of deep burns in radially oriented spots throughout the cornea (Fig. 2–7). These burns shrink the cornea periphery and increase the central corneal curvature (Fig. 2–8).

In 1898, Lans[14] first demonstrated the ability of superficial corneal burns to shrink tissue and change the refractive power of the cornea. Subsequently, this procedure was not further investigated until the late 1970s when it was used to treat keratoconus.[15–19]

In 1981, Fyodorov applied this concept to the correction of hyperopia in the form of radial burns and termed the procedure thermokeratoplasty.[20] With this procedure, a heat probe was used to perform 16 radial burns at a temperature of 600° C at 90% of corneal depth. These radial burns cause shrinkage and subsequent flattening in the periphery while steepening the central portion of the cornea.

Neumann's prospective evaluation of Fyodorov's 117 thermokeratoplasty eyes found that the technique reduced hyperopia from a mean of +5.27 diopters preoperatively to a mean of +1.84 diopters 12 months postoperatively with minimal regression. Other studies[21,22,23] have found similar amounts of undercorrection with this technique while experiencing greater amounts of regression. This regres-

sion has been speculated to be due to burn induced scars, even one year after the surgery, caused by the high temperature of the heat probe.

In order to increase the predictability of thermokeratoplasty, a new technique utilizing a holmium-YAG laser, instead of a heat probe, was first reported by Seiler in 1990.[21] With this new technique, infrared holmium-YAG laser light is delivered to the cornea in a series of spots placed in a cir-

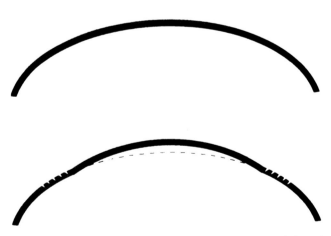

Fig. 2–8. Thermokeratoplasty resulting in peripheral weakening and central steepening.

cular pattern. The diameter of these spots is at least 5.0 mm and tightens the corneal periphery, creating a central steepening.[22,23] Seiler's initial data found hyperopic corrections up to 5.0 diopters with stability over the initial four months postoperatively. Subsequent studies[24,25,26] reveal a similar stability indicating that laser thermokeratoplasty may in fact be more predictable than thermokeratoplasty with a hot needle. Thermokeratoplasty using non-contact and contact techniques will be discussed by Drs. Vance Thompson, Douglas Koch and Antonio Mendez-Noble in this book. Recent studies using a variation of thermokeratoplasty with microwaves proved ineffective.[27]

KERATOPHAKIA AND KERATOMILEUSIS

Keratophakia and keratomileusis are refractive procedures that reduce hyperopia through the means of lamellar cuts. Jose Barraquer first proposed keratophakia and keratomileusis in 1961.[28,29,30] These techniques were introduced into the United States by Troutman and Swinger.[31]

With homoplastic keratophakia, a corneal lenticule cut from a donor cornea, frozen and shaped with a cryolathe into a refractive disk with central thickness.[32,33] Subsequently, a lamellar flap is made on the host cornea, the disk is inserted intrastomally, and the lamellar cut is replaced.

INTRACORNEAL LENSES

In reviews of this subject, Choyce[34] and Lane and Lindstrom[35] discussed their early work with fenestrated intracorneal lenses made of polysulfone as illustrated in Fig. 2–9. They reviewed the early work in this field which dates back to 1949. At that time, Barraquer originated the idea of placing intracorneal lenses made of flint glass (6 mm in diameter) and tested these lenses in rabbits and cats. Despite modifications and the use of other materials such acrylic, there was a loss of transparency with vascularization and extrusion of lenses.[36] Knowles suggested that the degeneration of the stroma and epithelium anterior to the intracorneal lenses was caused by interference with diffusion of metabolites and the selective desiccation of the corneal epithelium anterior to the lens. Epithelial integrity may be maintained by nutrients from the aqueous phase.[37]

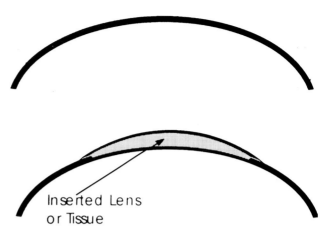

Fig. 2–9. Alloplastic keratophakia in which a manufactured lens is placed below the lamellar flap.

This led to the fenestration of polysulfone intracorneal lenses that led to better metabolic diffusion but a signficant number of nebular opacities.[35] A more recent approach includes the use of high water-content hydrogels.[38] These lenses allow diffusion of metabolites and are well tolerated. Intracorneal lenses will be discussed by Richard L. Lindstrom MD.

Hyperopic keratomileusis originally entailed removing a lenticule from the host cornea with a microkeratome, freezing the host lenticule and shaping it with a cryolathe to produce central thickness. The lenticule is then replaced. Results of this initial procedure varied primarily as result of tissue damage induced by the freezing process.[39–41] With the advent of the automated keratome,[42] Ruiz observed that a single, deep pass of the microkeratome could produce significant hyperopic correction without the need for using a lenticule.[43] This deep cut causes central corneal ectasia in the thinned tissue under the flap (Fig. 2–10). Studies on this technique are continuing[44,45] but progressive ectasia in a significant percentage of eyes makes this approach risky. David Hardten MD discusses his experience with ALK for hyperopia and the problems of progressive ectasia.

CLEAR LENS EXTRACTION

Intraocular lens correction of hyperopia has also joined with cataract technology to produce a surgical technique termed clear lens extraction for hyper-

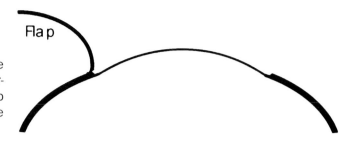

Fig. 2–10. Hyperopic ALK. A single, deep pass of the microkeratome could produce significant hyperopic correction without the need for using a lenticule. This deep cut causes central corneal ectasia in the thinned tissue under the flap.

opia. This procedure entails removing the normally functioning, noncataractous lens with phacoemulsification through a scleral tunnel. An IOL of the appropriate power is then inserted and placed in the capsular bag. This procedure was first reported for myopia by Fukala in 1889[46] and applied to hyperopia by Lyle and Jin in 1994.[47] This and subsequent studies[48–49] provide encouraging possibilities for correcting high degrees of hyperopia with the safety and precision of cataract technology. Isfahani and Salz will discuss clear lens extraction.

EXCIMER LASER

The most recent procedure for correcting hyperopia is with the use of the excimer laser termed hyperopic photorefractive keratectomy, called H-PRK. The principle of hyperopic correction with the laser was first proposed by L'Esperance in 1983.[50,51]

With this technique, a 193 nm argon fluoride (ArF) excimer laser beam is used to ablate superficial tissue and create a central corneal steepening, resulting in a more hyperopic eye (Fig. 2–11). Similar work was done with the early prototypes of the VISX laser. The Taunton LV 2000 excimer laser, pictured in Fig. 2–12, an early prototype excimer laser had a rotating series of apertures with an expanding central area which shielded the center of the cornea and allowed for a peripheral ablation (Fig. 2–13). Sher et al in 1991[52] described a technique using the Taunton LV 2000 excimer laser in which a peripheral steepening using the laser is performed after the central cornea is treated to remove scars. This technique, called a "unity cut" reduced the amount of hyperopic shift seen after the central cornea is treated. A similar technique can be performed with the Summit excimer laser by using a masking agent such as methylcellulose in the central cornea.

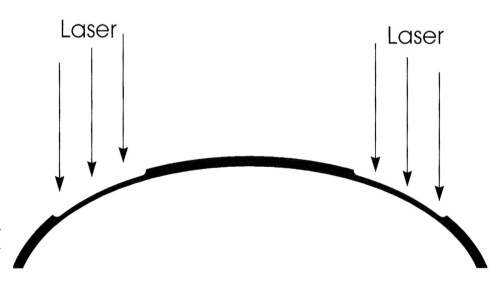

Fig. 2–11. Hyperopic laser correction with peripheral tissue ablation.

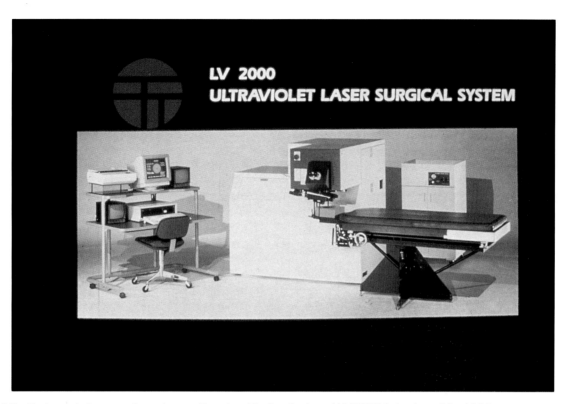

Fig. 2–12. Early prototype excimer laser, Taunton Technologies, LV 2000 introduced in 1989.

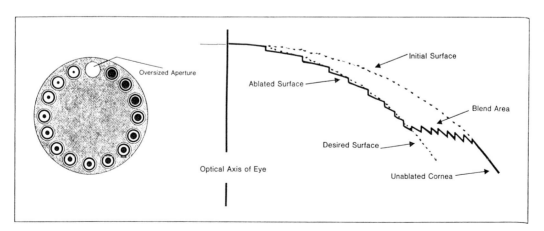

Fig. 2–13. Schematic of hyperopic correction wheel in Taunton Technologies LV 2000. Series of apertures with expanding central masked area steepened peripheral cornea.

The mechanism for ablating the peripheral tissue varies with laser manufacturers. Techniques for peripheral ablation range from wide area ablations with central corneal sparing to scanning slit, flying spot, blocking agents, and masks. Clinical investigations of PRK with hyperopia were initiated in 1991 by Dausch, Klein and Anschutz and reported in 1993.[53] This report corrected fifteen low hyperopic eyes (+2.00 to +7.50 D) to +0.53 diopters and eight highly hyperopic eyes (+11.00 to +16.00 D) to +2.5 diopters. Regression between one and nine months was +0.7 diopters for the low group and +3.0 diopters for the high group. Anschutz[54] acquired similar data in reports of 81 hyperopic eyes.

Regression of effect, undercorrection and a higher complication rate presents the greatest problem to the effectiveness of hyperopic PRK. Deep ablations created in the periphery of highly hyperopic patients induce epithelial hyperplasia and other healing patterns that reduce predictability. Postoperative haze is also more of a problem with hyperopic PRK than with myopic PRK. H-PRK will be discussed by Dausch, Lawless, Kraff, Sutton, Swinger.

LASIK has also been advocated for hyperopia. LASIK avoids the problems of epithelial hyperplasia and is believed to control some of the healing problems associated with hyperopic PRK. Hyperopic LASIK include cutting a flap in a small diameter and flat cornea and the need for a larger ablation zone. Klaus Ditzen MD will present his data on hyperopic LASIK.

SUMMARY

This chapter has reviewed the numerous surgical techniques, attempted over the last 100 years to treat hyperopia and presbyopia. A number of procedures have been tried and abandoned due to a variety of problems. The study of these past investigations and failures is very valuable in choosing the best approaches to this problem. Presently, there is no procedure that has gained wide acceptance and much research remains to be done.

REFERENCES

1. Bores LD: *Refractive eye surgery.* Boston, Blackwell Scientific, 1993.

2. Akiyama K: Study of surgical treatment for myopia. I. Posterior corneal incisions. *Acta Soc Ophthalmol Jpn* 56:1142, 1952.

3. Yamashita T, Schneider ME, Fuerst DJ, Pearce WJ: Hexagonal keratotomy reduces hyperopia after radial keratotomy in rabbits. *J Refract Surg* 2:261–264, 1986.

4. Gills J: Trephination in combination with radial keratotomy for myopia. In Schachar R, et al.: Radial Keratotomy. LAL, Dennison, 1980.

5. Neumann AC, McCarty GR: Hexagonal keratotomy for correction of low hyperopia: Preliminary results of a prospective study. *J Cataract Refract Surg* 14:265–269, 1988.

6. Mendez A: Hexagonal keratotomy for hyperopia. *Proceedings of the Keratorefractive Soc,* New Orleans, 1986.

7. Basuk WL, Zisman M, Waring GO 3rd, et al: Complications of hexagonal keratotomy. *Am J Ophthalmol* 117:37–49, 1994.

8. McDonnell PJ, Jean JS, Schanzlin DR: Globe rupture from blunt trauma after hexagonal keratotomy. *Am J Ophthalmol* 103:241–242, 1987.

9. Jensen RP: Hexagonal keratotomy. Clinical experience with 483 eyes. *Int Ophthalmol Clin* 31:69, 1991.

10. Pinsky PM, Datye DV: Numerical modeling of radial, astigmatic, and hexagonal keratotomy. *Refract Corneal Surg* 8:37–49, 1992.

11. Gilbert ML, Friedlander MH, Granet N: Corneal steepening in human eye bank eyes by combined hexagonal and transverse keratotomy. *Refract Corneal Surg* 6:126–130, 1990.

12. Grandon SC, Sanders DR, Anello RD, et al: Clinical evaluation of hexagonal keratotomy for the treatment of primary hyperopia. *J Cataract Refract Surg* 21:140–149, 1995.

13. Nordan LT, Maxwell WA: Avoid both keratotomy with small optical zones and hexagonal keratotomy. *Refract Corneal Surg* 8:331, 1992.

14. Lans LJ: Experimentelle Untersuchungen uber die Entstehung von Astigmatismus durch nicht-perforierende Conreawunden. *Graefes Arch Clin Exp Ophthalmol* 45:117–152, 1898.

15. Aquavella J: Thermokeratoplasty. *Ophthalmic Surg* 4:39–48, 1976.

16. Gasset AR, Schaw EL, Kaufman HE, et al: Thermokeratoplasty. *Trans Am Acad Ophthalmol* 77:441, 1973.

17. Kennas R, Dingle J: Thermokeratoplasty for keratoconus. *Ophthalmic Surg* 6:89–92, 1975.

18. Shaw EL, Gasset AR: Thermokeratoplasty (TKP) temperature profile. *Invest Ophthalmol Vis Sci* 13: 181–186, 1974.

19. Gasset AR, Kaufman HE: Thermokeratoplasty in the treatment of keratoconus. *Am J Ophthalmol* 79:226–232, 1975.

20. Newmann AC, Sanders D, Raanan M, DeLuca M: Hyperopic thermokeratoplasty: Clinical evaluation. *J Cataract Refract Surg* 17:830–838, 1991.

21. Seiler T, Matallana M, Bende T: Laser thermokeratoplasty by means of a pulsed holmium: YAG laser for hyperopic correction. *Refract Corneal Surg* 6:328, 1990.

22. Schachar RA: Radial thermokeratopasty. *Refract Surg* 3:47, 1990.

23. Moreira H, Campos M, Sawusch MR, et al: Holmium laser thermokeratoplasty. *Ophthalmology* 100:752–761, 1993.

24. Seiler T, Matallana M, Bende T: Leserkoagulation der Hornhaut mit einem Holmium: YAG-Laser zur Hyperopiekorrektur. *Fortschr Ophthalmol* 88:121–124, 1991.

25. Durrie DS, Schumer DJ, Cavanaugh TB: Holmium: YAG laser thermokeratoplasty for hyperopia. *J Refract Corneal Surg* 10:S277–280, 1994.

26. Thompson VM, Seiler T, Durrie DS, Cavanaugh TB: Holmium: YAG laser thermokeratoplasty for hyperopia and astigmatism: An overview. *Refract Corneal Surg* 9:S134–137, 1993.

27. Rowsey JJ: Electrosurgical keratoplasty: Update and retraction. *Invest Ophthalmol Vis Sci* 28 (suppl):224, 1987.

28. Barraquer JI: Queratoplastia. *Arch Soc Am Oftalmol Optom* 3:147–168, 1961.

29. Barraquer JI, ed: *Queratoplastia Refractiva*. Vol 1. Bogota, Colombia, Instituto Barraquer de America, 1970.

30. Barraquer JI. Keratomileusis for the correction of myopia. *Ann Inst Barraquer* 5:209–229, 1964.

31. Troutman RC, Swinger C: Refractive keratoplasty: Keratophakia and keratomileusis. *Trans Am Ophthalmol Soc* 76:329–339, 1978.

32. Friedlander MH, Rich LF, Werblin TP, et al: Keratophakia using preserved lenticules. *Ophthalmology* 87:687–692, 1980.

33. Maguen K, Pinhas S, Verity SM: Keratophakia with lyophilized cornea lathed at room temperature. *Ophthalmic Surg* 14:759–762, 1983.

34. Choyce DP: Intra-cameral and intra-corneal implants. A decade of personal experience. *Trans Ophthalmol Soc UK* 86:507–525, 1966.

35. Lane SS, Lindstrom RL: Polysulfone intracorneal lenses. *Int Ophthalmol Clin* 31:37–46, 1991.

36. Barraquer JI: Modification of refraction by means of intracorneal inclusions. *Int Ophthalmol Clin* 6:53–78, 1966.

37. Knowles WF: Effect of intralamellar plastic membranes on corneal physiology. *Am J Ophthalmol* 51: 1146–1156, 1961.

38. McCarey BE, Andrews DM: Refractive keratoplasty with intrastromal hydrogel lenticular implants. *Invest Oph Vis Sci* 21:107–115, 1981.

39. Schanzlin DJ, Jester JV, Eunduck K: Cryolathe corneal injury. *Cornea* 2:57–68, 1983.

40. Swinger CA, Krumeich J, Cassiday D: Planar lamellar refractive keratoplasty. *J Refract Corneal Surg* 2:17–24, 1986.

41. Binder PS, Zavala EY, Baumgartner SD, et al: Combined morphological effects of cryolathing and lyophilization on epikeratoplasty lenticules. *Arch Ophthal* 104:671–679, 1986.

42. Hofmann RF, Bechara SJ: An indepedent evaluation of second generation suction microkeratomes. *J Refract Corneal Surg* 5:348–354, 1992.

43. Ruiz LA: *Lamellar Keratectomy for hyperopia.* Kerato Refractive Society, Dallas, 1987.

44. Hollis S: Hyperopic lamellar keratoplasty. In Rozakis GW, ed: *Refractive Lamellar Keratoplasty.* Thorofare, Slack, 1994.

45. Manche EE, Judge A, Maloney RK: Lamellar keratoplasty for hyperopia. *J Refract Surg* 12:42–49, 1996.

46. Fukala V: Surgical treatment of high degrees of myopia through aphakia. *Graefes Arch Ophthalmol* 36:230–244, 1890.

47. Lyle WA, Jin GJ: Clear lens extraction for the correction of high refractive error. *J Cataract Refract Surg* 20:273–276, 1994.

48. Obstbaum SA: Clear lens extraction for high myopia and high hyperopia. *J Cataract Refract Surg* 20:271, 1994.

49. Siganos DS, Siganos CS, Pallikaris IG: Clear lens extraction and intraocular lens implantation in normally sighted hyperopic eyes. *J Refract Corneal Surg* 10:117–124, 1994.

50. L'Esperance FA Jr: *Ophthalmic Lasers,* ed 2. St. Louis: Mosby-Year Book, 1989:892.

51. L'Esperance FA Jr, Warner JW, Telfair WB, et al: Excimer laser instrumentation and technique for human corneal surgery. *Arch Ophthalmol* 107:131–139, 1988.

52. Sher NA, Bowers RA, Zabel RW, Frantz JM, Eiferman RA, Brown DC, Rowsey JJ, Parker P, Chen V, Lindstrom RL: The Clinical Use of the 193 nm Excimer Laser in the Treatment of Corneal Scars. *Arch Ophthalmol* 109:491–498, 1991.

53. Dausch D, Klein R, Schroder E: Excimer laser photorefractive keratectomy for hyperopia. *J Refract Corneal Surg* 9:20–28, 1993.

54. Dausch D, Landesz M: The Aesculap-Meditec Excimer Laser: Results from Germany. In Salz JJ, ed: *Corneal Laser Surgery.* St. Louis, Mosby, 1995.

section II

Incisional and Suture Techniques

CHAPTER 3

The Correction of Hyperopia Using Suture Techniques: Use of the Grene Lasso for Reduction of Hyperopia Following Radial Keratotomy

R. Bruce Grene

INTRODUCTION

The problem of hyperopia following radial keratotomy (RK) surgery has become of increasing concern since the discovery of a small but significant percentage of patients experiencing progressive hyperopia following RK.[1,2] Reports by Werblin suggest a stabilization of this progressive hyperopia.[3] Spigelman and Lindstrom suggest ("mini") improved stability with minimal RK procedures.[4] Nonetheless, the estimate of potential patients at risk for progressive hyperopia ranges as high as 100,000 patients (based upon an estimated 1,000,000 patients having undergone radial keratotomy over the past decade). This represents a significant public health risk and demands that refractive surgeons address safe and effective means of dealing with post radial keratotomy hyperopia. Fig 3–1 shows a case of post RK overcorrection which requires therapy

Even in the absence of progressive hyperopia, radial keratotomy, as with all incisional refractive procedures, bears an element of unpredictability due to variations in wound healing. A small but significant percentage of patients heal with wound gape. This means that even patients undergoing minimal RK procedures are at risk for the complications of post RK hyperopia. This complication is associated with both irregular astigmatism and overcorrection.[5,6] The cycle of wound gape leading to irregular astigmatism and overcorrection is shown if Fig. 3–2 (Grene's Triad). Fig. 3–3 represents a decision making tree when overcorrection is present.

The historical therapeutic options for dealing with iatrogenic hyperopia include spectacles, contact lenses and additional refractive surgery procedures. Spectacles are generally poorly tolerated in the presence of induced hyperopia. Life-long myopes are loathe to adapt to plus spectacles lenses. In addition, spectacle lenses do little to minimize the ghosting and blur of irregular astigmatism induced by post-RK wound gape.

Although contact lenses can now be fit with great consistency following radial keratotomy, soft contact lenses do little to ameliorate the induced irregular astigmatism. All contact lens material may aggravate fluctuations in corneal hydration, making visual fluctuation worse. The use of rigid gas permeable (RGP) contact lenses offers the best optical solution for both the induced hyperopia, as well as the irregular astigmatism associated with overcorrected radial keratotomy. Unfortunately, many patients are intolerant of RGP lenses either due to discomfort or due to conflicts related to work or vocational activities.

The frustrations experienced by surgeons and patients alike have led to a number of refractive surgical techniques being developed for the treatment of post radial keratotomy hyperopia. The use of automated lamellar keratoplasty (ALK) was popularized recently. Unfortunately, the use of a corneal transecting technique (which depends upon controlled ectasia), is fraught with additional problems when performed in patients who have a proven defect in corneal wound healing. In an effort to avoid these more invasive surgical procedures, surgeons have utilized a variety of suture compression techniques to reduce both the wound gape and to reverse the change in corneal shape induced by radial keratotomy.

The use of interrupted sutures has declined due to the difficulty in adjusting suture tension evenly among numerous individual sutures. In addition, asynchronous wound healing leads to the removal of interrupted sutures at different rates and to the occurrence of induced irregular astigmatism. Circumferential or purse string sutures have been used to equalize corneal compression.[7,8] The majority of

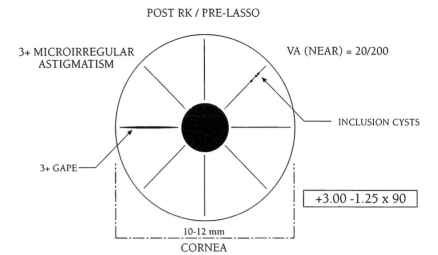

Fig. 3–1. Fig. 3–1 shows a case of post RK overcorrection which requires therapy.

reports describe intrastromal purse string sutures. A recent long-term follow-up reported by Lyle and Jin show generally good results in a population of 13 eyes of 12 patients.[9] The intrastromal suture techniques generally require retrobulbar anesthesia, are time consuming, and are somewhat limited in their effect due to the uniplanar nature of intrastromal suture passage.

In an effort to create an improved corneal suture technique for the reduction of hyperopia following radial keratotomy, the author developed a modifi-

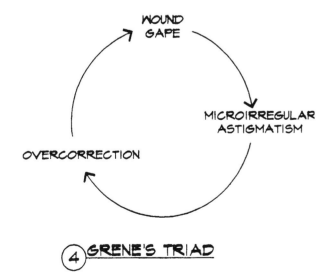

Fig. 3–2. Grene's Triad.

cation of the purse string suture. This modification involves a change in the suture path in order to both compress gaped RK incisions, and to reverse the knee created by RK surgery [Fig. 3–4 Lasso Technique]. The sinuous path of the Grene Lasso suture conveys significantly more posterior force to flatten the radial keratotomy knee. This aspect of the Grene Lasso variation allows a virtually unlimited amount of central corneal steepening. Fig. 3–5 shows a patient 30 days postop with a Grene Lasso suture.

The mechanism of effect of the Grene Lasso can be most easily demonstrated by observing the corneal power changes documented by intraoperative topography. Fig. 3–6A and 3–6B shows a typical PAR topography. As demonstrated in the topography images, the initial central flattening is effectively reversed. The areas of dark purple represent isolated regions of marked corneal depression. These regions correlate to the surface passage of the suture over the top of the gaped radial keratotomy incisions.

Through the use of the Grene Lasso compression suture, patients can experience significant improvement in their distance and near uncorrected visual acuity. Although the procedure (as with all corneal suture compression techniques) is expected to be temporary, patients have been enthusiastic about the visual benefit and the relief from symptoms from iatrogenic hyperopia.

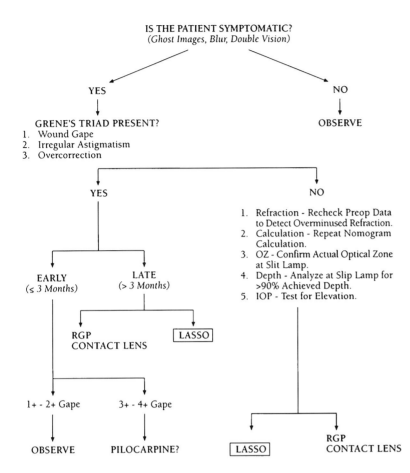

IS THE PATIENT SYMPTOMATIC?
(Ghost Images, Blur, Double Vision)

YES   NO

GRENE'S TRIAD PRESENT?   OBSERVE
1. Wound Gape
2. Irregular Astigmatism
3. Overcorrection

YES   NO

                                                       1. Refraction - Recheck Preop Data
      to Detect Overminused Refraction.
2. Calculation - Repeat Nomogram
      Calculation.
3. OZ - Confirm Actual Optical Zone
      at Slit Lamp.
4. Depth - Analyze at Slip Lamp for
      >90% Achieved Depth.
5. IOP - Test for Elevation.

EARLY   LATE
(≤ 3 Months)   (> 3 Months)

RGP   LASSO
CONTACT LENS

1+ - 2+ Gape   3+ - 4+ Gape

OBSERVE   PILOCARPINE?   LASSO   RGP
                                                CONTACT LENS

Fig. 3–3. Decision making tree for patients with overcorrection.

CURRENT SURGICAL TECHNIQUE

Criteria for Patient Selection

Prior to surgery, patients undergo a thorough preoperative ophthalmologic evaluation. Distance and near best corrected and uncorrected acuities are obtained. Manual keratometry is performed with careful attention to estimates of irregular astigmatism. Corneal topographic imaging is carried out with calculation of the mean central five millimeters keratometric value. A slit lamp exam is performed with attention to the estimation of wound gape. Fig. 3–7A is a slit lamp photograph of the incision and Fig. 3–7B shows the guidelines for estimating wound gape as well as a slit lamp estimation of incision depth. A refraction is performed using fogged manifest technique. Slit lamp photography is per-

formed as indicated. Following extensive discussion of the benefits, risks, and limitations of the procedure, patients who elect to proceed with surgery are scheduled. Surgery is always performed on a unilateral basis.

Current Surgical Technique

Surgery is generally performed in an outpatient ambulatory refractive surgery center. Topical anesthesia is applied. The patient is placed under the operating microscope and an initial intraoperative topographic study performed (PAR Corneal Topography System—PAR Vision Systems Corp., New Hartford, NY). In the absence of intraoperative topography, preoperative topographic images are obtained and the suture tension adjusted after postoperative images are obtained. Alternatively, pre-

GRENE LASSO: TECHNIQUE

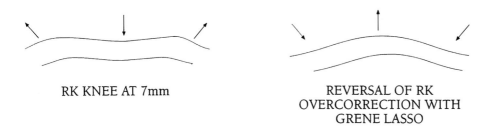

RK KNEE AT 7mm   REVERSAL OF RK
                                  OVERCORRECTION WITH
                                  GRENE LASSO

TRADITIONAL CONTINUOUS SUTURE TECHNIQUE   GRENE LASSO

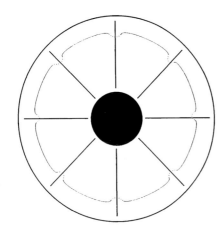
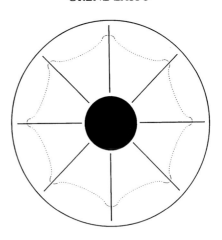

Fig. 3–4. Traditional Suture Technique + Lasso Suture Technique.

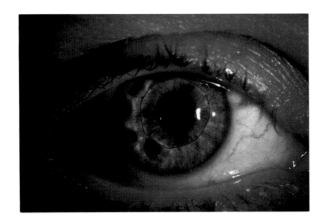

Fig. 3–5. Grene Lasso suture, 30 days postop.

and postoperative keratometry readings can be used if topography is unavailable.

A central visual axis mark is made and the 7 mm optical zone marker is used to make an impression (without ink) in the corneal epithelium. The surgical microscope is then turned to a low power of illumination. A gentle indentation is made at the limbus to help visually identify the location of previously placed radial keratotomy incisions. A modified needle specially designed for this procedure is utilized (Ethicon Modified CSB6). A variety of suture materials have been utilized, but the author currently recommends either 10-0 Nylon or 9-0 Nylon as the suture material of choice.

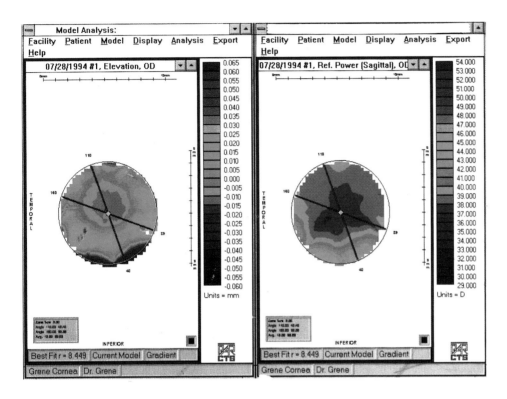

Fig. 3–6A. Par Topography photo, preoperative.

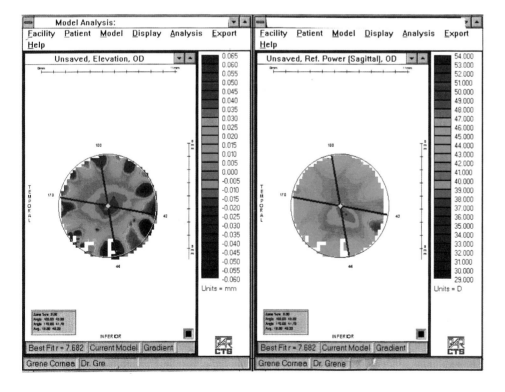

Fig. 3–6B. Par Topography photo postoperative.

pass over each radial incision. For previous 16- and 4-incision RK, 8 lasso bites are placed. For 6- and 3-incision RK, 6 stromal passes are made. A triple throw is made and laid flat on the corneal surface. A lid speculum is temporarily removed and another intraoperative corneal map is made. The suture is then adjusted based upon the desired corneal steepening. The preoperative mean central corneal keratometry value (for the central 5 mm region) is compared to the desired mean K-value. The suture is then tightened or loosened and a final image taken to assure that the appropriate amount of corneal steepening has been induced.

Fig. 3–8A–D shows a typical case. In the case presented, the evolution of corneal curvature is clearly displayed. The preoperative image (8A) shows the excessive central flattening characterized by blue colors for both corneal power and relative elevation. The initial check of corneal shape change (8B) shows the the lasso has induced macroirregular astigmatism and that the suture tension is uneven. Fig. 3–8C shows an improved symmetry, but the sutre is too taut as evidenced by the mean K of 48 D. Fig. 3–8D shows excellent symmetry and achieves the desired six diopters of central steepening. A one diopter regression is expected.

If intraoperative topography is unavailable, then the patient may be removed from the operating suite and taken to a testing area for topography or keratometry measurements, then returned to the operating room. After the new corneal power has been determined, three additional throws are made to create a secure knot. The author has observed postoperative regression of 1 diopter in nearly all cases. Therefore, it is recommended that the suture is tied when the desired amount of steepening **PLUS** one diopter, has been reached. If the desired result is a mean K of 42 D, then the keratometric reading immediately postop should be 43 D. The suture is then gently rotated so that the knot moves underneath the stromal surface. Suture tension is adjusted by gently pushing on each exposed loop of suture with a Y-hook. Topical analgesic (Ketorolac Acular™, Allergan Pharmaceuticals), and antibiotic (Ocuflox™, Allergan Pharmaceuticals) are applied. Both Celluvisc™ and Refresh Plus™ (Allergan Pharmaceuticals) are applied frequently during the procedure in order to both protect the ocular surface and to maintain sufficient optical clarity to

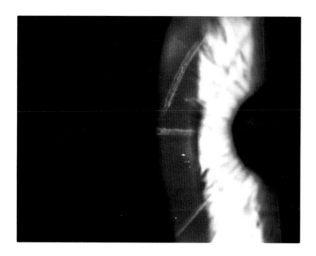

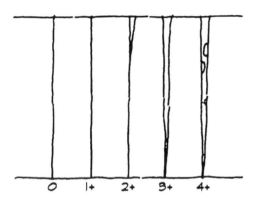

O - THIN LINE, AS IF DRAWN W/ SHARP PENCIL

I+ - THICK LINE, AS IF DRAWN W/ DULL PENCIL

2+ - ANTERIOR "SNAKE TONGUE" GAPE

3+ - FULL LENGTH GAPE

4+ - FULL LENGTH GAPE WITH PSEUDOCYSTS

Fig. 3–7. Wound gape photo and companion drawing.

The needle is gently rotated through the stroma to approximately 80% depth. Each bite is placed between the previous radial keratotomy incisions. The suture passes over each radial incision. This is the only section of suture which is exposed to the corneal surface. For a previous 8-incision RK, the lasso will make eight intrastromal bites and

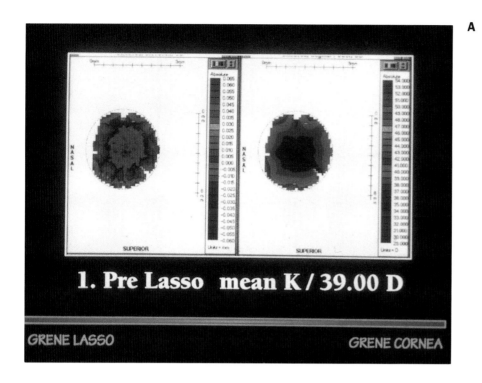

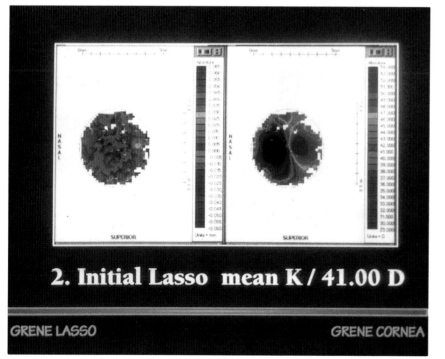

Fig. 3–8A,B. PAR case study: In the case presented, the evolution of corneal curvature is clearly displayed. The preoperative image (8A) shows the excessive central flattening characterized by blue colors for both corneal power and relative elevation. The initial check of corneal shape change (8B) shows the the lasso has induced macroirregular astigmatism and that the suture tension is uneven.

(continued)

C

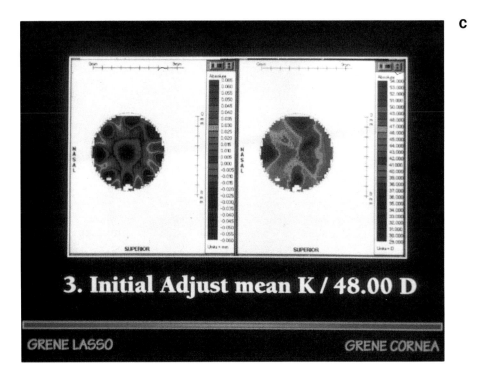

D

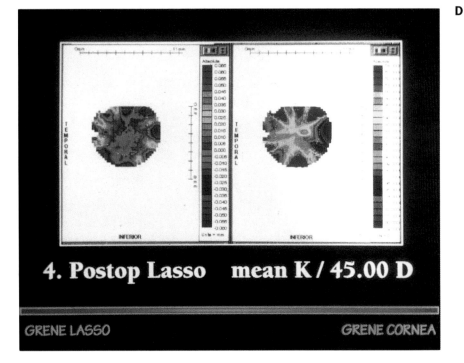

Fig. 3–8C,D. Figure 8C shows an improved symmetry, but the suture is too taut as evidenced by the mean K of 48 D. Figure 8D shows excellent symmetry and achieves the desired six diopters of central steepening. A one diopter regression is expected.

allow intraoperative topographic images to be accurately captured.

Postoperative Management

The immediate medical management includes topical analgesic (Acular™, Allergan Pharmaceuticals), topical antibiosis (Ocuflox™, Allergan Pharmaceuticals), and topical steroid (1% prednisolone acetate Pred Forte™, Allergan Pharmaceuticals). The antibiotic is generally utilized q.i.d. for five days. Both the topical analgesic and topical steroid are titrated depending upon the amount of observed cornea inflammation and patient symptoms. It is common to taper these medications gradually over two to three months based upon office examinations every two to four weeks.

The patient is generally seen at one day and two weeks, and monthly thereafter. It is important that patients be counseled to return **immediately** should they experience foreign body sensation or symptoms of increased photophobia, pain, or tenderness. At approximately two-to-four weeks, it is possible to determine whether the lasso suture is too tight or too loose. Sutures that are slightly too loose can be easily tightened using an anchor suture technique.[9] Sutures which are judged to be significantly too tight may need to be replaced or lengthened.

Surgical Results

The visual results of 85 lasso procedures performed in a population of 68 patients are presented. The preoperative mean spherical equivalent was + 2.01 diopters. The postoperative mean spherical equivalent was reduced to + 0.07 diopters. This resulted in an improvement in mean distance acuity from 20/50 to 20/40. Near vision improved from 20/80 uncorrected acuity to 20/30 uncorrected near acuity.

A number of patients underwent multiple procedures, including replacement, adjustment or anchor sutures. Of the 68 patients undergoing 85 procedures, 66 eyes required one to two procedures. Nineteen eyes required three or more procedures.

Complications

The risks associated with the lasso suture technique parallel that of any other corneal suturing technique. These risks include infection, undercorrection, overcorrection and suture breakage. An additional unexpected complication has been seen with the lasso technique. We have noted an unusually high incidence of inflammatory keratitis. Unlike interrupted sutures and intrastromal sutures, the Grene Lasso technique appears to have a higher than expected incidence of inflammatory keratitis with the attendant symptoms of photophobia, pain and tenderness. This inflammation can lead to "cheese-wiring" and in rare cases, perforation. To minimize these risks, we strongly favor nylon suture. In addition, we favor a longer surface suture passage to increase support and minimize "cheese-wiring". This necessitates a short stromal bite for which the modified CSB-6 needle was developed (Ethicon).

SUMMARY

The challenge of surgical reduction of hyperopia remains one of the last frontiers in refractive surgery. The Grene Lasso is one of several evolving procedures for the treatment of hyperopia following radial keratotomy. The advantages of the Grene Lasso technique over other suture techniques include its greater power and its greater simplicity of placement. The advantages of this suture technique over nonsuture techniques include both its adjustability and removability. The disadvantages of the Grene Lasso stem from an unacceptable incidence of inflammatory keratitis. We estimate that one in three patients have some form of reaction in the first year. However, we have discontinued using Prolene and Mersilene, and now use nylon suture material exclusively. Our early experience with nylon suture indicates much greater stability.

In addition, it must be recognized as a temporary correction because the technique depends upon a suture for effect. The Grene Lasso technique for reduction of hyperopia has a valuable role in our refractive surgery armamentarium. Continued improvements in the technique may allow a greater acceptance by refractive surgeons and patients alike. Certainly, the treatment of all forms of hyperopia remains a great challenge, and we look forward to the development of superior surgical techniques in the future.

REFERENCES

1. Deitz MR, Sanders DR, Raanan MG, Deluca M: Long-term (5–12 year) follow-up of metal-blade radial keratotomy procedures. *Arch Ophthalmol* 112: 614–620, 1994.
2. Waring GO, Lynn MJ, McDonnell PJ, et al: Results of the prospective evaluation of radial keratotomy (PERK) study 10 years after surgery. *Arch Ophthalmol* 112:1298–1308, 1994.
3. Werblin TP, Stafford GM: The Casebeer system for predictable keratorefractive surgery: one year evaluation of 205 consecutive eyes. *Ophthalmology* 100: 1095–1102, 1993.
4. Spigelman AV, Williams PA, Nichols BD, Lindstrom, RL: Four incision radial keratotomy. *J Cataract Refract Surg* 14:125–128, 1988.
5. Grene RB: How to reduce induced hyperopia. *Rev Ophthalmol* March 1995: 86–89.
6. Sanders D, Deitz M, Gallagher D: Factors affecting predictability of radial keratotomy. *Ophthalmology* 92:1237–1243, 1985.
7. Waring GO: Refractive Keratotomy for Myopia and Astigmatism. St. Louis, Mosby Year Book, 1992.
8. Starling JC and Hofmann RF: The new surgical technique for the correction of hyperopia and radial keratotomy: Experimental model. *J Refract Surg* 2:9–14, 1986.
9. Lyle WA and Jin GC: Long-term stability of refraction after intrastromal suture correction of hyperopia following radial keratotomy. *J Refract Surg* 11:485–489, 1995.

CHAPTER 4

Anterior Ciliary Sclerotomy (ACS), A Procedure to Reverse Presbyopia

Spencer P. Thornton

INTRODUCTION

Presbyopia has become the new frontier of refractive surgery. Though it eventually affects everyone, few are happy with the consequences. Many see it as a sign of advancing age, and feel that it is a handicap in many activities.

It is estimated that new cases of symptomatic presbyopia—that is, cases that require reading glasses or bifocals—approach three million per year in the United States. Couple this with the number of older individuals who are unhappy with their current reading glasses or bifocals, and the number of potential candidates for a presbyopia reversing procedure becomes astronomical.

In the early 1980s we learned that carrying radial incisions past the limbus into the anterior sclera produced a lessening of the desired effect of corneal (RK) incisions. For example, if four diopters of effect had been predicted by nomogram and the incisions were carried past the limbus into the anterior sclera, 25 to 30% less effect was obtained than predicted, with a resulting undercorrection of a diopter or so. The full effect was only obtained when the incisions stopped short of the limbus.

Other problems, such as bleeding during the RK procedure, regression of effect and subsequent ingrowth of vessels onto the cornea along the incision lines, led to the abandonment of RK incisions crossing the limbus into the anterior sclera. Regression of effect became less frequent. On the other hand, progression of effect (gradual hyperopic shift) was soon noted, leading to the observation that the globe is a dynamic structure with a delicate balance of responses to surgical alteration.

Though the mechanism of action is not fully understood, the principle of globe circumference enlargement by surface incisions has been demonstrated clinically in radial and astigmatic keratot-

omy for a number of years. The limitation of the globe's increased circumference to the cornea when incisions are confined within the limbus is felt to be due to the "barrier effect" of the circumferential ligament of the cornea, located at the limbus. This same barrier prevents corneal alteration when incisions are made peripheral to the limbus in anterior ciliary sclerotomy.

As noted above, the reduction of hyperopia and myopic shift seen with anterior ciliary sclerotomy is not new. What was a problem—and a complication—in the early 1980s, appears to be the solution to a problem of the late 1990s—presbyopia.

THE PRINCIPLE OF ANTERIOR CILIARY SCLEROTOMY

Anterior Ciliary Sclerotomy is based on the theory of accommodation proposed by Cramer in 1860 and reported by Donders in 1864.[1] Cramer held that accommodation resulted primarily from ciliary body contraction with resulting forward movement of the lens. Though his theory was virtually discarded by his contemporaries in favor of the "relaxed zonules with altered lens curvature on ciliary contraction" theory, recent re-evaluation of the evidence has confirmed the anterior movement of the lens-zonule complex on accommodation.[2]

The underlying rationale of Anterior Ciliary Sclerotomy is based on the observation that the lens is ectodermal in origin and constantly grows throughout life, gradually "crowding" the posterior chamber and eventually preventing full function of the ciliary body/zonular complex. Rather than a loss of elasticity of the lens with age, it is felt that this "crowded" state is the cause of the reduction of lens power change with attempted accommodation.

33

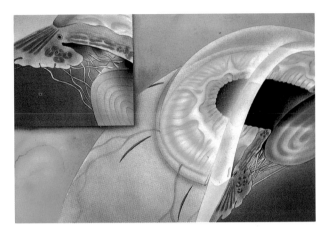

Fig. 4–1. Theoretical mechanism of ACS. The natural expansion of the lens with aging may result in loose zonules [insert], which are put on stretch with the expansion of the scleral diameter.

If the ciliary body is impaired in its ability to move or change the shape of the lens because it is "crowded" by the lens, then making more room for the ciliary body would allow more space for the lens-zonule complex. By expanding the globe in the area of the ciliary body this could be accomplished.

THE ANTERIOR CILIARY SCLEROTOMY TECHNIQUE

The ACS procedure involves no implanted bands or suturing. It is an incisional technique. There is no difference in principle in the action of incisions in the sclera from that of incisions placed in the

peripheral cornea—i.e., radial incisions increase the circumference at right angles to the direction of the incisions and produce a peripheral "knee" or bulge in the cornea.[3] Thus if the scleral incisions are radial, the globe will increase in circumference over the ciliary body, creating more room for the muscle, and consequently more room for the lens and zonules. If the ciliary muscle and lens-zonule complex are otherwise normal, the provision of more space should provide more normal accommodative action. See Figures 4–1, 4–2 and 4–3.

The ACS procedure is the isolation of one part of the RK procedure as it was done in the early 1980s, tailoring it to a specific application. What was undesirable with RK is now seen to be desirable for the purposes of reversal of RK overcorrection and potential restoration of accommodative amplitude lost with presbyopia.

Current Surgical Technique

The technique involves placing eight symmetrical partial-thickness radial incisions into the sclera over the ciliary body to allow an expansion of the sclera and resulting increase in scleral diameter over the ciliary body. This allows an increased area for ciliary muscle action and consequent increased zonular effectiveness in changing the focal power of the lens. The use of only four incisions results in reduced effect. More incisions produce more effect. Both refractive and age-related nomograms are being developed.

The ACS procedure can be enhanced or reversed. Enhancement is achieved by adding more incisions, and reversed by suturing previously placed incisions.

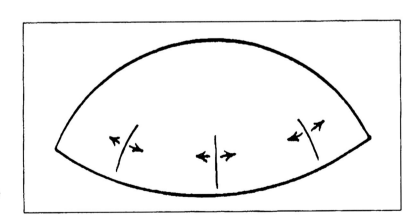

Fig. 4–2. Radial incisions increase the globe's circumference.

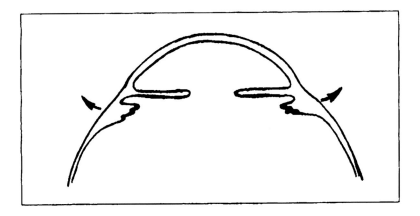

Fig. 4–3. Incisions over the ciliary body increase the scleral diameter.

The recommended technique consists of eight partial-thickness, mini-radial incisions over the ciliary body in the anterior sclera beginning one millimeter back from the limbus (the point at which the iris can no longer be seen through cornea) and carried two and a half millimeters posteriorly, over the ciliary body, stopping just anterior to the pars plana. The desired incision depth is approximately 65 to 70% (diamond micrometer blade set at about 450 microns), stopping when the ciliary body can be seen through the sclera or when the scleral tissue begins to spread. Either steel or diamond blade may be used. For greater effect the procedure can be titrated by adding up to eight more incisions any time after placement of the original eight.

Our original approach was to perform a circumferential perilimbal peritomy to expose the peri-limbal sclera. Another approach is to place four radial incisions through the bulbar conjunctiva and tenons at 12, 3, 6 and 9 o'clock, with blunt dissection under this opened peri-limbal conjunctiva to allow this opening to be pulled to one side and then to the other so that eight radial scleral incisions can be made through only four conjunctival incisions. When finished, the conjunctival incisions do not overlay the scleral incisions, making the eye more comfortable and reducing the chance of infection.

Another approach, used by several investigators, is the trans-conjunctival approach (diamond micrometer blade setting about 650° to allow for the increased thickness of conjunctiva and tenons), preceded by careful Betadine prep of the bulbar conjunctiva. In this approach the incisions are made beginning one millimeter posterior to the anatomic limbus (the point at which the iris is no longer visi-

ble through the cornea) and carried 2.5mm posteriorly, being sure to stop short of the pars plana.

POTENTIAL COMPLICATIONS

Potential complications of ACS include infection, hemorrhage (from cutting too deep), ocular hypotension, myopic shift (possibly from change in axial length), and compromise of the limbal conjunctival barrier. In patients who are hyperopic, any myopic shift is a "reduction of hyperopia" and an additional benefit rather than a complication.

The possibility of perforation through the pars plana demands careful attention to anatomic landmarks to avoid carrying the incisions past the ciliary body into pars plana. The incisions must be limited to the sclera over the ciliary body to obtain maximal effect. Also, if you perforate posterior to the ciliary body, there is the risk of retinal detachment. Perforation anteriorly carries the risk of peripheral iris injury or prolapse.

PREOPERATIVE EVALUATION

Accurate determination of postoperative effect must begin with accurate pre-operative assessment.

In the Informed Consent, the patient must be informed that Anterior Ciliary Sclerotomy is a "non standard procedure", and "an investigational procedure".

The preoperative assessment must include:

1. Manifest and cycloplegic refraction: Manifest refraction should be done in normal room

lighting (not dimmed). The pupil diameter must be noted for post-operative comparison to maintain an equivalent depth of focus.

2. Measure the accommodative amplitude by near chart and Prince rule.

3. Measure axial length by A-scan to determine if the myopic shift seen in early reports may be due to change in the axial length or position of the lens.

4. EyeSys Topography to determine the possibility of enhanced focal range by limbal flattening and/or increased asphericity.

SUMMARY

The traditionally held view that presbyopia is caused by an age-related loss of elasticity of the lens has been challenged by the theory that it is the result of a continually growing lens with a reduction in the space between the lens capsule equator and the cil- iary body which is restricted by a non-growing sclera. With this reduced range of action, the ciliary body is limited in its ability to alter the shape or position of the lens on attempted accommodation. By placing partial thickness incisions in the sclera over the ciliary body, the globe is expanded in that area, allowing greater ciliary action and consequent greater accommodation.

REFERENCES

1. Donders, FC: On the Anomalies of Accommodation and Refraction of the Eye. London, The New Sydenham Society, 1864. pp 25–26 (translated by William Daniel Moore).

2. Thornton, S: Lens implantation with restored accommodation. *Curr Can Ophthalmic Prac.* 4:2, June, 1986.

3. Thornton, S: Astigmatic Keratotomy: A Review of Basic Concepts. *J.Cataract Refract Surg* 16:27–31, July 1990.

section III

Photoablation for Hyperopia and Presbyopia

A. Excimer Laser

CHAPTER 5

Excimer Laser Photorefractive Keratectomy (PRK) for Hyperopia: Aesculap-Meditec—North American Experience

Peter Stockdill

INTRODUCTION

Aesculap-Meditec is a pioneer in the treatment of hyperopia, with the first experimental studies being carried out in 1990. Aesculap-Meditec GMBH, Heroldsberg, Germany, has been developing and manufacturing medical laser systems since 1977. The first model for photorefractive keratectomy, the MEL 50, was introduced in 1986. Since then, the machine has been upgraded to the MEL 60 and several hundred have been installed worldwide. The first MEL 60 excimer laser in Canada was installed at the Mitchell Eye Centre in Calgary, Alberta in August 1994. Since then, four more of these lasers have been installed in Canada. In addition to these lasers, there are four Aesculap-Meditec MEL 60 lasers in Mexico, and four more have just been installed in the United States to undergo the FDA clinical studies. When initially installed, these lasers used a hyperopic treatment mask with a 7.5 mm ablation zone and a 4 mm optical zone. At the present time, the trend is to upgrade all Aesculap-Meditec excimer lasers to use the new hyperopic treatment mask with a 9.0 mm ablation zone and a 6.0 mm optical zone.

HISTORICAL REVIEW OF CURRENT TECHNIQUE

The Aesculap-Meditec MEL 60 laser is a 193 nm (ArF) laser with a frequency of 20 Hz and a fluence of 250 mJ/cm2. The Meditec MEL 60 excimer laser uses a rotating treatment mask and a scanning slit beam (10 × 1 mm) to sculpt the cornea into the shape required for the correction of hyperopia. This involves ablating the more peripheral areas of the cornea and avoiding the central area so that a convex surface can be created in the optical zone. The central portion of the cornea is guarded by the mask permitting the treatment of the more peripheral areas by the laser (Fig. 5–1). See Figures 6–1 through 6–4 for photographs of laser system.

One of the advantages of the Aesculap-Meditec concept is the use of the treatment masks and handpieces. This enables the manufacturer to alter the treatment method by redesigning the treatment mask without necessitating consequential major changes to the laser delivery system itself.

As an example of this, the original hyperopic treatment mask was a rotating spiral mask (Fig. 5–2). This mask was replaced in 1993 by a totally redesigned treatment mask with a 7.5 mm ablation zone (Fig. 5–1) to permit successful treatment of hyperopic patients requiring up to 7 diopters of correction.

Early studies using this technology began to point out difficulties with the higher hyperopic corrections. It was generally felt that larger optical zones and larger ablation zones were necessary for satisfactory results in patients with greater than 5 diopters of hyperopia.[1] Because of significant regression in the attempted correction of hyperopia over 7 diopters, a new hyperopic treatment mask using a similar design, but a 9.0 mm ablation zone with a 6 mm optical zone, was developed by Aesculap-Meditec and introduced in 1995 (Fig. 5–3).

The combination of the rotating treatment mask and the scanning laser beam that is integral to the Aesculap-Meditec technology ensures a smooth surface and smooth transition zones.[2] The second generation mask can also be used for the simultaneous correction of hyperopic astigmatism.

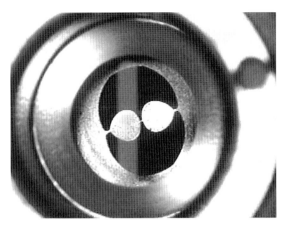

Fig. 5–1. Surgeon's view of the Meditec 7.5mm hyperopic treatment mask. The red helium-neon (He-Ne) beam operates coaxially with the excimer laser. During treatment, the mask rotates and the He-Ne/Excimer beam scans back and forth.

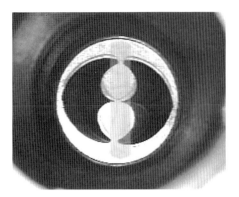

Fig. 5–3. Surgeon's view of the Meditec 9mm hyperopic treatment mask. The red helium-neon (He-Ne) beam operates coaxially with the excimer laser. During treatment, the mask rotates and the He-Ne/Excimer beam scans back and forth.

The Aesculap-Meditec MEL 60 uses a suction ring to hold the eye during the procedure and the hyperopic mask is placed within this ring during treatment (Fig. 5–4). Surgeon fixation using this suction device is essential to ensure accurate centration of the ablation. Because of its scanning technology, the MEL 60 laser takes more time to complete a treatment than the full area ablation lasers, and thus patient fixation is more difficult. The convex nature of the correction required in hyperopia necessitates accurate centration to a greater degree

than in myopia in order to avoid glare and halo problems as well as poor visual results.[3,4]

CURRENT SURGICAL TECHNIQUE

General Considerations

The hyperopic patient seeking PRK correction tends to be much older than the average myopic patient. Although we see an age group that includes

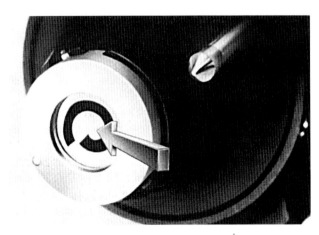

Fig. 5–2. Original Meditec hyperopic treatment with spiral-shaped aperture.

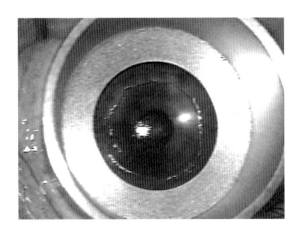

Fig. 5–4. Meditec suction ring in place following removal of the epithelium. Note the centration.

20 and 30-year old patients seeking myopic corrections, the hyperopic patients tend to be aged 40 to 75. This brings forward a number of issues that will be discussed in the next section.

The matter of unilateral vs. simultaneous bilateral treatment is an issue for all PRK surgeons, but when one is treating hyperopic patients, additional issues must be considered as compared with the myope.[5]

The hyperopic patients tend to be older than the myopic ones, and there may be additional general health factors impacting on the healing of their eyes. The ablation zone is much larger than for most myopic corrections and so the healing time is several days longer. In addition, the return of vision is much slower after a hyperopic correction and so patients who do undergo bilateral treatment must be advised that they may not be able to drive for several weeks.

Criteria for Patient Selection

Patients are not selected only on the basis of a refractive error that the surgeon feels can be successfully corrected. As in myopic corrections, certain patients should be excluded from treatment (Table 5–1). This includes those who are pregnant, have an unstable refractive error, systemic autoimmune disease or active ocular disease, severe diabetes or a history of poor wound healing. Patients with a pacemaker are not treatable because of electromagnetic energy which can be radiated from the laser power supply and cause disruption in the operation of the pacemaker.

Table 5–1. Contraindications for Photorefractive Keratectomy

- Severe dry eye or blepharitis and meibomianitis
- Pregnancy
- Keratoconus
- Proliferative diabetic retinopathy
- Systemic autoimmune disease (e.g., systemic lupus erythematosus or rheumatoid arthritis)
- Cataract
- Glaucoma
- History of herpetic keratitis
- Corneal neovascularization
- Cardiac pacemaker
- Unrealistic expectations

Due to the older age of the hyperopic PRK patients, more care is necessary preoperatively in assessing potential problems. Patients with severe dry eyes, blepharitis and meibomianitis should not be treated, or have their blepharitis and meibomianitis treated (including expressing the meibomian glands if indicated), before undergoing PRK. Care must be taken to exclude early cataracts or glaucoma.

As with the myopic candidate for PRK, the emotional condition of the patient must also be considered. Patients who hold unrealistic expectations from PRK are not good candidates, and the surgeon is wise to uncover this tendency early when establishing the suitability of the candidate.

Persons who have recently gone through an emotional event such as a divorce or death in the family should be advised to wait six to twelve months before proceeding with PRK.

Patient Objectives

It is important to uncover individual goals from the prospective patient. In other words, find out how they would define a successful outcome of their PRK treatment. Obviously they wish to see better without their glasses or contact lenses, but it is useful to the surgeon to find out the degree of improvement to their vision that is required in order for the patient to feel the procedure was successful.[6]

For some patients, the goal is to be able to see the alarm clock. Some patients require a certain line of vision for their profession. Others want to be able to see their children, for example, when woken in the middle of the night. I have had more than one patient who is motivated by what they refer to as a security factor. These patients travel extensively and are therefore frequently in an unfamiliar environment and want to be able to find exits without their glasses in the event of an emergency. In discussing goals with patients, I find asking them "How will we judge success?" a useful tool, and I record their answer in their chart for future reference.

Preoperative Management

At the time of initial consultation, all relevant risks and options are fully discussed with the patient. They must all be advised that reading glasses will be needed postoperatively, although my experience is that many of these patients can read sometimes without glasses. My patients are encouraged to bring along their spouse or close friend and it is at this time that both are informed that the success of the procedure will depend not only on the operation of the laser, but their cooperation in following postop instructions carefully. I have found that many PRK patients arbitrarily decide that postop drops are not really necessary and frequently the recommended postop medication schedule is not followed.

With time, I have learned that many of these PRK patients are different from the average "sick" patients that we have treated for years. These PRK patients are perfectly well, they just want to see more clearly without their glasses. Consequently, they need much more detailed and written instructions as to postoperative care and they have to be repeatedly reminded of these instructions. I find that informing a spouse or friend of the requirements is very helpful.[7]

All patients have a full ophthalmic examination. As part of this examination, the patient's pupil size is noted as patients with large pupils may experience halos and difficulty driving at night. A cycloplegic refraction is done on all hyperopes and this information is used for programming the laser. Corneal topography is carried out to screen for preclinical keratoconus and irregular astigmatism. If indicated, the axial length and corneal thickness are also measured.

SURGICAL PROCEDURE

Calibration of the Laser

The Aesculap-Meditec MEL 60 excimer laser uses a strip of special aluminium-coated test paper to check the fluence of the laser and the homogeneity of the laser beam before every patient is treated. The paper is red in color. As the aluminium is ablated by the laser, the red color should appear after nine scans of the laser (Fig. 5–5). The power of the laser can be adjusted and the calibration test repeated until the operator is assured that the fluence level is correct and the beam is homogeneous. This calibration check is carried out within 15 minutes of every patient treatment.

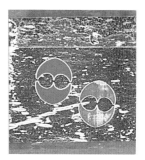

Fig. 5–5. Meditec fluence test paper, showing a correct calibration on the left and insufficient energy on the right. Note that some residual aluminum is on the test area.

The Procedure

All patients receive topical anaesthetic drops (proparacaine hydrochloride 0.5%), and in some cases ketorolac tromethamine 0.5% (Acular, Allergan) or diclofenac sodium 0.1% (Voltaren, Ciba Vision Ophthalmics) prior to treatment.

When ready, the patient is positioned under the laser, and the lid speculum is inserted. The center of the planned ablation is marked with a Sinskey hook and a suitable marker ring is used to define the area of epithelium to be removed. The epithelium is either removed manually or with the assistance of a few drops of 15% absolute alcohol which is placed within the ring for 15–30 seconds. This technique has been shown to have no impact on the refractive result.[8,9] In removing the epithelium, the central area is left until the end (to reduce dehydration). Regardless of the technique of removal, it is most important to remove the epithelium quickly and start the laser treatment immediately to avoid drying of Bowman's membrane and stroma.[10,11]

After removal of the epithelium, the center of the pupil is once again marked with the Sinskey hook. The suction ring holding device with its centering cross (Fig. 5–6) is placed in such a manner that the center of the cross is over the mark made by the Sinskey hook. The surgeon applies suction to the ring by pressing a foot switch and when there is adequate vacuum in the system, (0.3–0.4 bar) the centering cross is removed.

The hyperopic handpiece with its rotating treatment mask is then placed inside the suction ring.

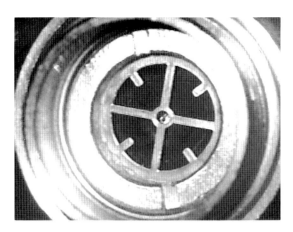

Fig. 5–6. Centering cross within the suction ring. The small central round opening is placed over the center mark on the cornea made by the Sinskey hook. Note the edge of the epithelium.

The handpiece is rotated so that the long solid axis of the treatment mask is located along the 180 degree meridian. The laser beam is centered on the treatment mask and the laser is activated with a foot switch. During the treatment, the surgeon ensures that the scanning beam is always covering the opening in the treatment mask as it rotates. The position of the beam can be controlled by the surgeon using a joy stick on the arm rest of the chair.

With completion of the treatment, a drop of unpreserved artificial tears is placed on the cornea as a masking agent, dried slightly, and the laser activated again for up to nine more scans to "polish" the surface.[12,13] This "polishing" technique removes projecting edges and irregularities in the cornea, and as a result, substantially less haze is reported.

Several of the Canadian Centers are using ice cold balanced salt solution before and after photorefractive keratectomy to reduce discomfort and reduce subepithelial haze.[14]

POSTOPERATIVE MANAGEMENT

Contact Lens vs. Patching

Most patients treated in North America have a bandage soft contact lens placed until the eye has reep-

ithelialized. It is interesting that in Europe there is currently a trend away from contact lenses to patching.[15] The fit of the contact lens is important, and PRK surgeons who are unfamiliar with the proper fit of a contact lens will find it useful to inform themselves in this area.

If there is any suggestion of a tight fitting lens, such as discomfort or injection of the eye, it should be replaced with a looser lens or removed entirely. The lens should also be replaced if there are significant deposits on it.

The observation that there seems to be fewer epithelial healing problems when a bandage contact is not used, and the fact that in some areas surgeons are moving away from the use of these lenses and returning to patching, suggests that improvements may be able to be made in the design and fit of contact lenses for PRK cases.

Pain Relief

Although the bandage soft contact lens is a major factor in pain relief, there are many other modalities that can be suggested to the patient. These patients are frequently photophobic (even indoors) and they should be urged to use sunglasses as required. I insist on my patients using an unpreserved tear drop on an hourly basis. This provides pain relief, and also may be a factor in preventing the concentration of preservatives and other chemicals underneath the contact lens. Ice bags used for 20 minutes every two hours are helpful to many patients.[16] I suggest that my patients use these modalities before using a mild analgesic or the nonsteroidal anti-inflammatory drug, (NSAID) that I have provided. I suggest minimizing the use of the NSAID to a maximum of every 6–12 hours at most, and only for the first 24–36 hours after their treatment. It has been shown that these drugs can slow down epithelial healing. In addition, NSAIDS have been implicated in the development of sterile post-operative corneal infiltrates.[17] It has been suggested that the concurrent use of a steroidal drop will reduce the incidence of these infiltrates. This may be so, but in my experience the steroid does not eliminate the occurrence of these infiltrates. It is also possible that the presence of a contact lens has some impact on the development of these infiltrates.

SURGICAL RESULTS

The following results are from a multicenter survey of hyperopia treatment using the Meditec excimer laser in Canada. Five centers were involved and approximately 15 surgeons. Data was not included unless there was at least three months of follow up. The attempted corrections ranged from +0.5 diopter to +7.0 diopters. The centers that submitted data to the study are listed in Table 5–2.

The mean refraction over time, is shown in Fig. 5–7. This graph shows a mean preoperative refraction of +3.1 diopters (range +1.0 to +6.0), reducing to 0.5 diopters (range −1.87 to +4.0) at three months and then regressing slightly at six months to a mean of +0.83 diopters (range −1.25 to +4.75). There is insufficient 12-month data to include in the study.

The scattergram at six months (Fig. 5–8) shows 69.7% of the cases within 1.0 diopter of the attempted correction. When one looks at those cases where the attempted correction was less than +4.0 diopters, 77.8% of these cases were within 1.0 diopter of the planned correction. Well-centered smooth ablations are evidenced in the topographical maps shown in Fig. 5–9 and Fig. 5–10.

With regard to uncorrected vision, we found that the mean uncorrected vision at three months was 20/40 and this improved to 20/30 at six months (Fig. 5–11). Mean best corrected vision at three months was 20/30 and at six months 20/25 (Fig. 5–12).

The excimer laser has been shown to be effective in treating under-corrected radial keratotomy

Table 5–2. Multi-Center Study Participants

Excimer Vision Treatment Center	Vancouver, British Columbia
Image Plus Laser Eye Centre	Winnipeg, Manitoba
Laser Medcare	Ottawa, Ontario
Mitchell Eye Centre	Calgary, Alberta
Northern Alberta Eye Institute	Edmonton, Alberta

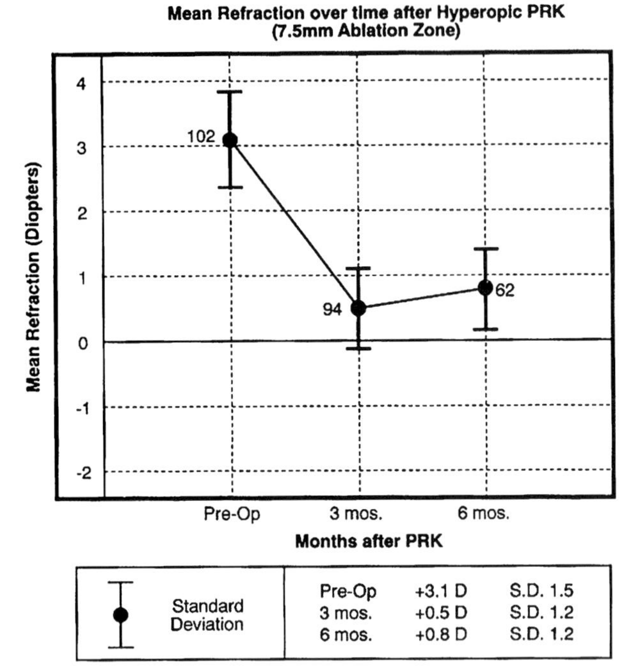

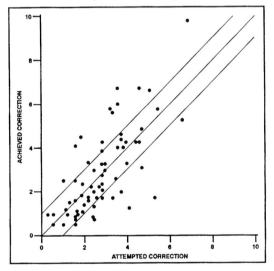

Mean Refraction over time after Hyperopic PRK
(7.5mm Ablation Zone)

		Pre-Op	
	Standard Deviation	Pre-Op +3.1 D	S.D. 1.5
		3 mos. +0.5 D	S.D. 1.2
		6 mos. +0.8 D	S.D. 1.2

Fig. 5–7. Mean manifest refraction (spherical equivalent) in diopters at various time intervals after hyperopic excimer PRK. The number adjacent to points represent the number of eyes at each data point.

Scattergram of Results 6 Months after Hyperopic PRK
(7.5mm Ablation Zone)

Fig. 5–8. Scattergram of attempted versus achieved correction at 6 months after hyperopic photorefractive keratectomy (spherical equivalent). Attempted corrections ranged from +0.5 to +7.0 diopters.

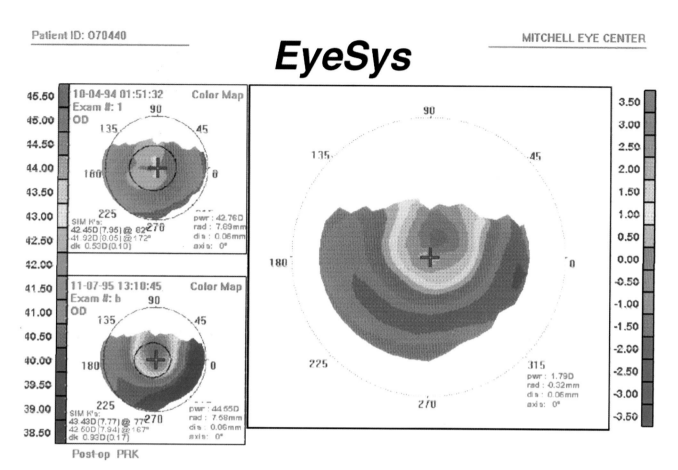

Fig. 5–9. Corneal topography map of a patient who had a preoperative refraction of +3.0 diopters. The preoperative map is on the top left and the 13 month postoperative map on the bottom left. The difference map is on the right. Note the well centered smooth ablation.

cases.[18,19,20] The Aesculap-Meditec excimer laser has also been shown to be very effective in treating patients who have been over-corrected by radial keratotomy. In a study recently presented, 23 patients aged 22–59 who were over-corrected after RK were treated and the results are shown in Fig. 5-13.[21] These patients (who had a mean preoperative refraction of +2.79 diopters), postoperatively had a mean refraction of −0.38 diopters. Many of these cases had been purposely made myopic. One eye did not respond to treatment, and some increased risk of haze was reported.

COMPLICATIONS

Complications in these cases have been relatively few in number. There were nine cases with postoperative refractions more than 2 diopters off the intended correction at six months. Two cases had significant haze and scarring and required retreatment.

One of the delayed healing cases took 20 days to heal and will require retreatment. The cause of the delayed healing is unclear, but was probably due to inadequate lubrication and a tight lens syndrome.

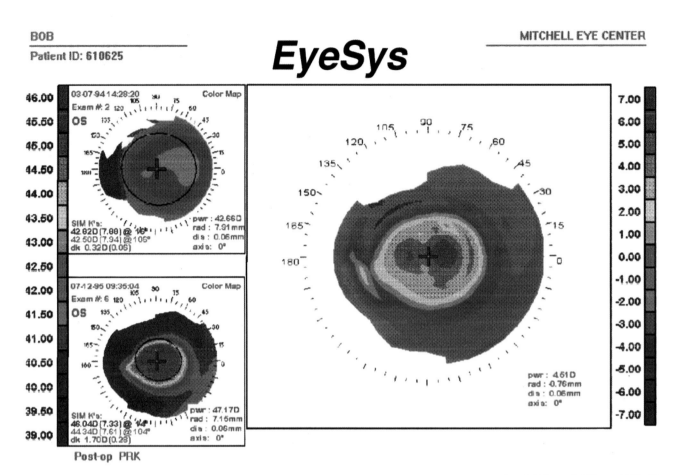

Fig. 5–10. Corneal topography map of a patient who had a preoperative refraction of +7.50 − 1.25 × 100. The preoperative map is on the top left and the 6 moth postoperative map on the bottom left. The difference map is on the right. Note the well centered smooth ablation.

UNCORRECTED VISUAL ACUITY			
	Pre-Op	3 Months	6 Months
Mean	20/150	20/40	20/30
Minimum		20/20	20/15
Maximum		20/100	20/100

Fig. 5–11. Uncorrected Visual Acuity at 3 and 6 Months.

BEST CORRECTED VISUAL ACUITY			
	Pre-Op	3 Months	6 Months
Mean	20/20	20/30	20/25
Minimum		20/20	20/15
Maximum		20/100	20/100

Fig. 5–12. Best Corrected Visual Acuity at 3 and 6 Months.

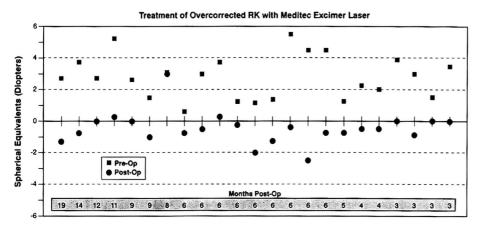

Fig. 5–13. Scattergram of results of 23 over-corrected RK eyes treated for their hyperopia with the Meditec Excimer laser. (Courtesy Dr. Jose J. de la Garza Viejo, Mexico).

The complications reported in this survey are shown in Table 5–3.

FUTURE PLANS AND DEVELOPMENTS

As previously stated, the trend in North America is to install the upgraded 9.0 mm hyperopic treatment mask in all Meditec excimer lasers. The results with this treatment modality are limited in North America, but results in Europe are most encouraging.

The Canadian results at three months with the 9.0 mm treatment mask are shown in Fig. 5–14. Although the numbers are very limited, they show

87.5% of cases within +/− 1 diopter of the intended correction. The mean preoperative refraction in these cases was +2.6 diopters and the attempted correction was less than +4.0 diopters in all cases.

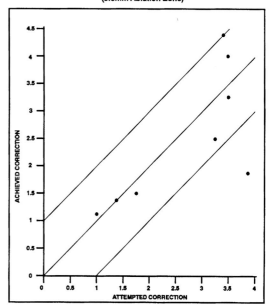

Fig. 5–14. Scattergram of attempted versus achieved correction (spherical equivalent) at 3 months after hyperopic photorefractive keratectomy using the 9.00 mm treatment mask at 5 Canadian centers.

Table 5–3. Complications

Complication	# of cases
Delayed healing of epithelium (more than 7 days)	1
Under/over correction (more than 2 diopters)	9
Sterile corneal infiltrates	0
Drug sensitivity	0
Glare and halos (after 3 months)	0
Haze and scarring (more than +1)	2
Other	0

The other developing area of interest is the Myopia 3 treatment mask which is used for the treatment of high and mixed astigmatism (Fig. 5–15). This treatment mask consists of an opening slit (5 × 9 mm) that is aligned along the axis of the minus cylinder. This slit gradually opens during the treatment producing a tapered edge to the ablation. The Myopia 3 treatment mask can be used in combined treatments with the hyperopic and myopic masks as shown in the topographic maps in Fig. 5–16 and Fig. 5–17. The early Canadian results in the treatment of hyperopic astigmatism with this technique are shown in Table 5–4.

SUMMARY

Canadian PRK surgeons using the Aesculap-Meditec MEL 60 laser and their patients are pleased with the results obtained so far in the treatment of hyperopia. However, some problems remain.

Epithelial healing remains a problem in some cases, and the reasons are not clearly established. The design and fit of the bandage contact lenses is

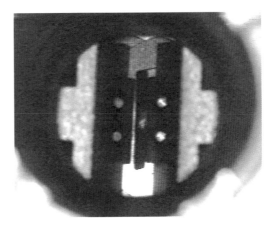

Fig. 5–15. Myopia 3 treatment mask used for the correction of pure astigmatism and mixed astigmatism. During treatment, the mask is positioned with the long axis aligned with the axis of the minus cylinder and the blades gradually open to a dimension of 9 × 5 mm.

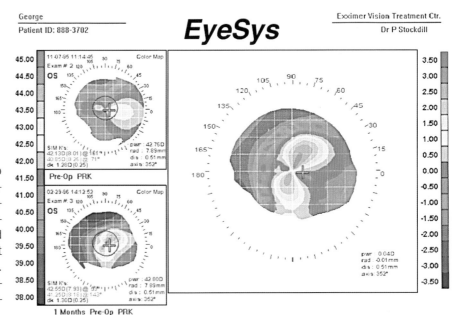

Fig. 5–16. Corneal topography map of the patient in Fig. 19. This patient was treated with a combination of the Myopia 3 and the hyperopic treatment masks. The pre and post-operative maps are on the left and the difference map on the right. This map was taken 1 month post-operative and shows a marked reduction in the astigmatism.

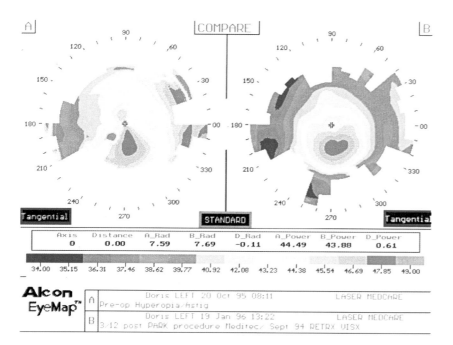

Fig. 5–17. Corneal topography map of a patient with a preoperative refraction of +2.50 − 4.00 × 10. The preoperative map is on the left and the 3 month postoperative map is on the right. Note the complete elimination of the astigmatism. This patient was treated with a combination of the Myopia 3 and the Hyperopic treatment masks. This patient had a PTK treatment in 1994 for a chemical burn scar. The eye was initially injured in 1967.

an area we may look to for improvements. The cause and prevention of sterile corneal infiltrates is still not clear and will require further investigation.

The results of the cases treated with the 7.5 mm ablation zone are very good up to about +4.0 diopters, but there is less accuracy with the higher corrections. European studies on the new 9.0 mm ablation zone for hyperopic treatment suggest there will be less regression and more accuracy, especially with the higher corrections. This is further sup-

ported by the early results of hyperopic cases that have been treated with the 9.0 mm ablation zone in Canada.

Haze was a major problem in the early studies of PRK. In this series, haze has been minimal (Figs. 5.18, 5.19). The exception occurred when there was a delay in epithelial healing. The reasons for this noticeable decrease in haze may be the smoother ablation pattern achieved with the Aesculap-Meditec laser, the use of the "polishing technique,"

Table 5–4. Early Canadian Results of Treatment of Hyperopic Astigmatism with Myopia 3 Mask

Patient	Follow up Time	Preop Refraction	Postop Refraction
DP	3 months	+2.50−4.00 × 10	+0.50
Note this patient had a previous PTK for a chemical burn in 1967.			
TM	3 months	+5.25−5.75 × 20	+5.25−4.75 × 30
Note this patient has had a previous perforating wound.			
MA	3 months	+1.50−2.50 × 90	−0.50−1.25 × 180
GN	1 month	+3.00−3.00 × 75	+2.00−2.00 × 10

Note this patient is age 75 and is pseudophakic

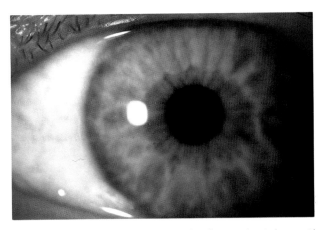

Fig. 5–18. Slit lamp photograph of a patient 1 month after PRK for a correction of +2.75 + 0.50 × 180. Note the clear cornea with minimal haze.

and perhaps the use of the cold balanced salt solution used right after the procedure.

Overall, excimer laser photorefractive keratectomy for hyperopia using the Aesculap-Meditec MEL 60 has established itself as a viable treatment, both with the surgeons and their patients. Continued study and the ensuing improvements in both technology and technique will, hopefully, further perfect this revolutionary procedure.

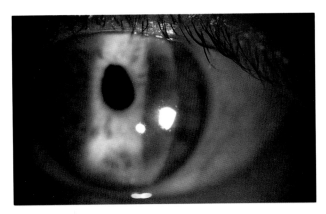

Fig. 5–19. Slit lamp photograph of a 74 year old pseudophake 1 month after PRK for a correction of +3.00 − 3.00 × 75. In spite of the fact that he has a few guttata, he has a clear cornea with no significant haze.

REFERENCES

1. Dausch D, Landesz M: *Corneal Laser Surgery*, St. Louis, Mosby, 1995, pp 238–241.
2. Dausch D, Klein R, Schroder E, Dausch B: Excimer laser photorefractive keratectomy with tapered transition zones for high myopia. *J Cataract Refract Surg* 19(5):590–594, 1993.
3. Dausch D, Klein R, Schroder E: Excimer laser photorefractive keratectomy for hyperopia. *Refract Corneal Surg* 9(1):20–28, 1993.
4. Maloney R: Corneal topography and optical zone location in photorefractive keratectomy. *Refract Corneal Surg* 6(5):590–594, 1990.
5. Machat J. Mintsioulis G: Unilateral vs. simultaneous bilateral photorefractive keratectomy. *Can J Ophthalmol* 30(4):181–182, 1995.
6. Stein H, Cheskes A, Stein R: *The Excimer Fundamentals and Clinical Use*. New Jersey, Slack, 1995, p 21.
7. Caubet E: Course of subepithelial corneal haze over 18 months after photorefractive keratectomy for myopia. *Refract Corneal Surg* 9(2 Suppl):S65–70, 1993.
8. Mendez-Noble A: Poster, American Academy of Ophthalmology, 1995, Atlanta, Georgia.
9. Stein H: Alcohol epithelium removal, presented at the Pacific Coast Refractive Symposium, Whistler, BC, Feb. 15–19, 1996.
10. Campos M, Trokel S, McDonnell P: Surface morphology following photorefractive keratectomy. *Ophthalmic Surg* 24(12):822–825, 1993.
11. Dougherty P, Wellish K, Maloney R: Excimer laser ablation rate and corneal hydration. *Am J Ophthalmol*, 118(2)169–176, 1994.
12. Azar D, Jain S, Woods K, et al: *Corneal Laser Surgery*. St. Louis, Mosby, 1995, p 215.
13. Aesculap-Meditec, PRK Polishing Bulletin, April, 1995.
14. Niizuma R, Hayashi M, Futemma M, et al: Cooling the cornea to prevent side effects of photorefractive keratectomy. *J Refract Corneal Surg* 10(2 Suppl):S262–266, 1994.
15. Schroder E: Personal communication.
16. Chayet A: The use of ice packs in the management of pain and discomfort following PRK. Presented at the Pacific Coast Refractive Symposium, Whistler, BC, Feb. 15–19, 1996.
17. Sher N, Krueger R, Teal P, et al: Role of topical corticosteroids and nonsteroidal anti-inflammatory

drugs in the etiology of stromal infiltrates after excimer photorefractive keratectomy. *J Refract Corneal Surg* 10(5):587–588, 1994.

18. Georaras S, Neos G, Margetis S, et al: Correction of myopic anisometropia with photorefractive keratectomy in 15 eyes, *Refract Corneal Surg* 9(2 Suppl): 29–34, 1993.

19. Hahn R, Kim J, Lee Y: Excimer laser photorefractive keratectomy to correct residual myopia after radial keratotomy. *Refract Corneal Surg* 9(2 Suppl):25–29, 1993.

20. McDonnell P, Garbos J, Salz J: Excimer laser myopic photorefractive keratectomy after undercorrected radial keratotomy. *Refract Corneal Surg* 7(2): 146–150, 1991.

21. Garza Viejo J: Experience in overcorrected eyes of RK treated with excimer laser, presented at the Pacific Coast Refractive Symposium, Feb. 15–19, 1996.

CHAPTER 6

Photorefractive Keratectomy for Hyperopia Aesculap-Meditec (German) Experience

Dieter Dausch
Z. Smecka
Robert Klein
Eckhard Schroeder

INTRODUCTION

Excimer laser photorefractive keratectomy for correcting hyperopia (H-PRK) was first performed by Dausch at al.[1,2] The results obtained with a 7 mm treatment zone, published in 1993, were good. However, when the method was applied clinically on a broader scale, high regression of the initial result occurred in isolated cases. Recent studies of myopic eyes after photorefractive keratectomy (PRK) suggest that a larger ablation zone may help resolve problems associated with PRK[3,4] with less variation in refractive outcome. Therefore we decided to enlarge the treatment zone for H-PRK also.

The following questions are relevant not only in the correction of myopia, but also for hyperopic-PRK:

1. Is the refractive outcome predictable?
2. Is the refraction attained stable?
3. Are there any complications or adverse reactions?
4. After five years experience is it time to ask if PRK is a suitable and effective tool for treating hyperopic eyes?
5. Does it represent a genuine alternative to other surgical methods?

This chapter discusses the clinical results of a study of 68 normally-sighted hyperopic eyes of 62 patients treated by PRK with an enlarged (9 mm) treatment zone.

CRITERIA FOR PATIENT SELECTION

Between January 1994 and January 1996, a total of 83 eyes of 75 patients (40 females, 35 males) underwent PRK to correct hyperopia. The mean age of the patients with 39.0 ± 11 years (range, 19 to 61 years). Preoperative refraction ranged from +2.00 D to +8.25 D. The BCVA for all eyes was 20/40 or better. Emmetropia was attempted in all cases.

Inclusion criteria stipulated that all patients should be at least 18 years of age and have a stable hyperopic spherical equivalent of +2.00 D or more. Candidates with more than 1.50 D of corneal cylinder were excluded. Other inclusion criteria mandated that both eyes be free of corneal scarring or diseases, severe dry eye symptoms, blepharitis and/or lagophthalmos. Exceptions were made for patients with micropannus secondary to long-term contact lens wear and mild lenticular changes consistent with the patient's age. Subjects with systemic disease were excluded. The therapy was discussed preoperatively with candidates who fulfilled the study criteria; the risks, side effects, possible complications, and alternative treatments were emphasized. The surgical technique used is described in the following section.

CURRENT SURGICAL TECHNIQUE

The excimer laser used in this study was a MEL 60, manufactured by Aesculap Meditec. (See Figs. 6–1 to 6–4). This laser emits energy with a wavelength of 193 nm. The exposures for large-area photoablation were performed with a repetition rate of 0.5 Hz. Each complete exposure was accomplished by a scanning process, not by a single illumination. To this end, the 9 × 1 mm slit profile was moved uniformly so that a rectangular area measuring 9 × 10 mm was exposed to the laser. (Fig. 6–5)

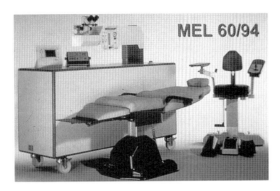

Fig. 6–1. MEL 60-94 Aesculap Meditec laser system (slide provided, print in B and W).

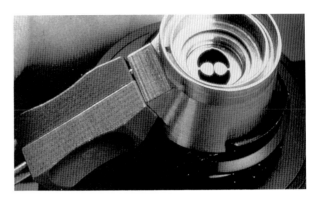

Fig. 6–4. Mask for correcting hyperopia, with a 9 mm aperture in the rotating template.

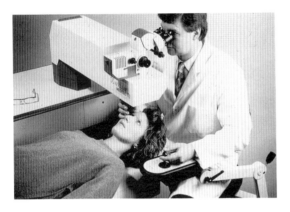

Fig. 6–2. Patient undergoing PRK with MEL 60-94 laser (slide provided, print in B and W).

Circular areas up to 9 mm in diameter can be treated in this way. The scan return points must be outside this area. The energy density of the individual laser beam was 250 mJ/cm^2, resulting in a corneal ablation depth of 0.5 mm per pulse. However, at a repetition rate of 20 Hz the scanning process was adjusted so that there was considerable overlap of adjacent laser shots. The total effect of one scanning process was therefore an ablation of 1 mm. This overlapping method also ensured that the ablation procedure produced smooth surfaces. The laser is controlled by a graphic display control panel. (Fig. 6–6).

The method used to correct myopia and hyperopia and the ablation profile for correcting hyper-

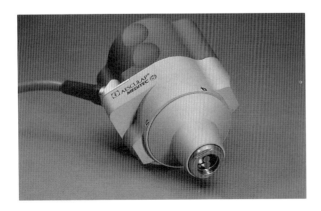

Fig. 6–3. MEL 60-94 computer controlled handpiece.

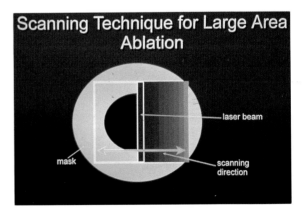

Fig. 6–5. Schematic of scanning.

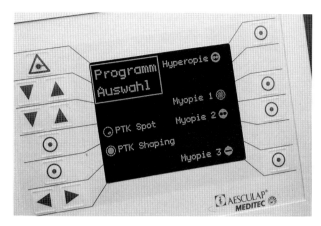

Fig. 6–6. MEL 60-94 control panel.

opia has been described elsewhere.[1,2,5] No ablation was performed in the central corneal region (0.3 to 0.5 mm in diameter); the greatest ablation depth was at the border of the treated area. However, since a steep excision border was not permissible, a transition zone was required that extended beyond the area corrected.

The ablation profile was altered using a rotating mask with a specially shaped aperture. The hyperopic mask has the special aperture in the rotating template. (Fig. 6–3, 6–4). In this case, the diameter of the corrected zone is 6 mm. The diameter of the total area ablated, including the transition zone, is 9 mm. The mask is inserted in a suction ring fixed on the patient's eye. The laser passes over the aperture after each angular increment. If the mask rotates regularly through 360°, symmetrical tissue ablation occurs, with the highest degree of steepening at the center. This enables spherical hyperopia to be corrected.

PREOPERATIVE MANAGEMENT

Preoperative measurements relevant to this study included uncorrected visual acuity and best spectacle-corrected visual acuity. Refraction, with and without cycloplegia, was performed prior to surgery in all patients. Keratometer readings (Zeiss-Ophthalmoskop, manufactured by Zeiss, Oberkochen, Germany) autorefraction (Humphrey model 515, manufactured by Humphrey, San Leandro, CA), visual acuity under glare conditions (Humphrey

model 515) and a slit lamp examination were performed. IOP was measured by Goldman applanation tonometry preoperatively and at every follow-up visit after one month. The severity of postoperative subepithelial haze was graded by two examiners according to the classification by Dausch, Klein and Schroder.[1,5]

SURGICAL PROCEDURE

The ablations were performed by two surgeons (Dausch and Smecka) using the same type of excimer laser. The homogeneity of the beam profile within the central 7 mm was better than 95%. The homogeneity and the ablation rate were calibrated with Afga L 720 RC photographic paper prior to each procedure.

The data for this clinical series were gathered prospectively, with postoperative examinations at days one, two, and three and at months one, three, six, nine and twelve. Refractive, keratometric, and visual acuity data were also obtained at these visits. Computer-assisted videokeratography (Corneal Modeling System [CMS], Computed Anatomy, Inc., New York, NY) was performed at all visits after surgery and cycloplegic refraction at the final visit.

The attempted correction for each eye was equal to the mean spherical equivalent corrected to the corneal plane determined from the manifest refraction obtained by two independent observers. Attempted corrections ranged from +2.00 to +8.50 D. The maximum ablation depth in Bowman's layer and the corneal stroma was approximately 115 μm.

The center of the ring-shaped excimer ablation was determined by marking the entrance pupil as the patient fixated on the light of the operating microscope. During the ablation procedure, the eye was stabilized by means of the mask and the suction ring. Other preoperative, operative, and immediately postoperative methods have been described elsewhere.[5]

Postoperative Management

Gentamicin ointment was applied postoperatively in all eyes until the epithelial defect healed. For the first month postoperatively, fluorometholone 0.1%

eyedrops were instilled five times daily. Subsequently, the dose was reduced by one drop per month during the next four months.

Surgical Results

One-month data were available on 83 eyes, three-month data on 79, six-month data on 77, nine-month data on 65, and 12-month data on 68. Mean values are presented with one standard deviation error bar. In the statistical analysis are 68 eyes that could be followed for up to one year. The data on the three eyes who lost the nine-month follow-up were comparable to the data of the other eyes who had all follow-up visits and were therefore included in the study.

Refraction

The time course of refraction is presented in Fig. 6–7: the mean spherical equivalent was +4.85 ± 1.85 D preoperatively. At one month this value averaged −0.63 ± 1.04 D, at three months −0.10 ± 1.13 D, at six months +0.29 ± 1.07 D and at 12 months +0.45 ± 1.16 D. The mean change from 1 to 12 months (one-year regression) was 1.08 D.

The distribution of individual spherical equivalent refraction at 12 months after PRK shows the consistency of the results (Fig. 6–8). After 12 months the spherical equivalent of 55 of 68 eyes (81%) was

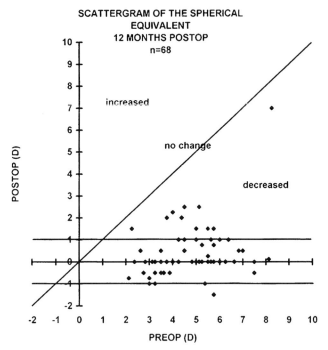

Fig. 6–8. Attempted versus achieved correction (diopters) at 12 months postoperatively.

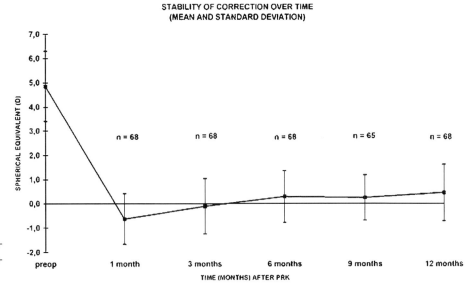

Fig. 6–7. Mean spherical equivalent (diopters) at various postoperative internals.

within ± 1.00 D. Thirteen eyes were outside this range and all except one were undercorrected. The spherical equivalent of 40 eyes (59%) was within ±0.50 D.

The changes in (manual) keratometer readings were significantly less marked than the changes in manifest refraction. They were of limited value and are not presented here. Also, the autorefractor readings indicated persistent hyperopia in some cases and were inconsistent with the manifest refraction.

Visual Acuity

Best spectacle corrected visual acuity ranged preoperatively from 20/63 to 20/16 (mean 20/25), decreasing slightly to a mean of 20/32 (range 20/63 to 20/20) at one month. At three months, the mean best spectacle corrected visual acuity was 20/25. At 12 months it remained 20/25. Four eyes (6%) lost one Snellen line, one eye (1%) lost two lines, and one eye (1%) lost three lines; 38 eyes (56%) showed no change and 24 eyes (36%) improved. The overall best spectacle corrected visual acuity at various intervals postoperatively is shown in Fig. 6–9.

To evaluate the efficacy of PRK for correcting hyperopia it is important to measure uncorrected visual acuity. The mean uncorrected visual acuity improved from 20/80 preoperatively to 20/32 at three months. At 12 months, 66 (97%) of eyes

treated had an uncorrected visual acuity of 20/40 or better, 27 eyes (40%) were 20/20 or better.

Topographic Results

Both direct and subtraction videokeratographic pictures were used to study the ablation profile. In all cases a circular steepening was found in the central cornea. A typical finding is shown in Fig. 6–10.

Centration was good in all but two of the eyes, which showed a decentration of 0.5 mm and 1.0 mm respectively. This correlated clinically with the loss of best corrected visual acuity. Four eyes showed a slight corneal irregularity in the central 3 mm. These cases also lost best corrected visual acuity.

COMPLICATIONS

Haze

The location of haze following H-PRK has some special features. In all cases the central cornea, including Bowman's layer, remained intact and clear. The haze formed a ring in all treated eyes. It was most dense at the border of the ablated zone. As in myopic PRK, all treated eyes had transient mild haze at one month. This haze disappeared completely within three to six months.

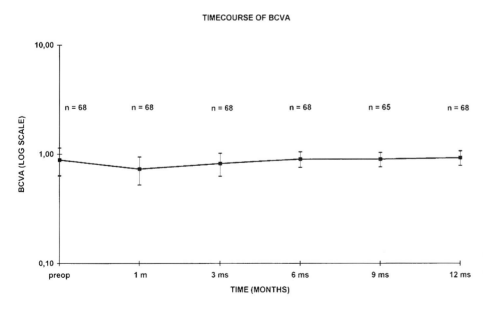

Fig. 6–9. Overall mean postoperative best corrected visual acuity at various postoperative intervals.

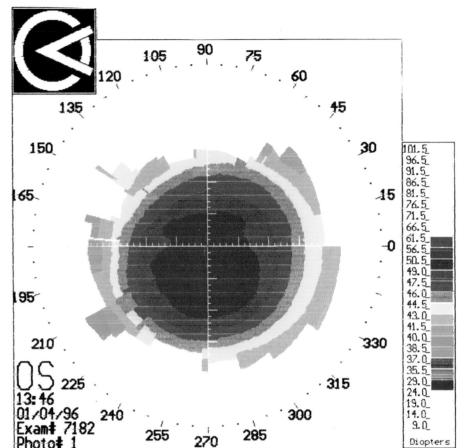

Fig. 6–10. Videokeratograph of an eye in which correction of 5.25 D was attempted. UCVA was 20/160. BCVA prior to surgery was +5.25 −0.75 × 104° = 20/20. The videokeratograph shows the status 12 months after PRK. The newly created clear zone, including transition zone, is visible as red-brown, red, and yellow areas. Manifest refraction 12 months postoperatively was plano; UCVA was 20/20.

Epithelial Disorders

In all cases the epithelial defect healed within three to six days. All 83 eyes healed without complications.

Intraocular Pressure

No increase in intraocular pressure of more than 3 mm Hg was seen in any eye at any visit.

Subjective Symptoms

All patients reported ocular pain during the 24 hours following surgery. Almost all complained of halos immediately after surgery. At six months, eight patients reported halos, albeit of diminished intensity, when driving at night. At 12 months none of the patients noticed persistent halos.

One month after surgery, six patients complained of glare. After one year only two patients reported this side effect.

DISCUSSION

In this chapter we presented a study of 68 sighted human eyes followed for 12 months after excimer laser PRK for hyperopia. All eyes had a best spectacle corrected visual acuity (BSCVA) of 20/40 or better. The results show that hyperopic eyes can be treated successfully with PRK. The mean preoperative spherical equivalent of +4.85 ± 1.45 D was reduced to −0.63 ± 1.04 D at four weeks postoperatively.

Safety

With regard to safety, loss of BSCVA and vision-threatening complications should be studied.

BSCVA was either improved or unchanged in 62 (92%) of the eyes. Four eyes (6%) had lost one line, one eye (1%) 2 lines and one eye (1%) 3 lines after 12 months. The reduction in best corrected visual acuity by two and three lines in two eyes may be related to a slight decentration of the treatment zone (0.5 and 1.0 mm) revealed by videokeratography. Loss of BSCVA by one line in four eyes may be explained by an irregular surface of the central cornea. Cases with corneal irregularity achieved an improvement in BSCVA by fitting a hard contact lens.

The time course of BSCVA at various postoperative intervals clearly shows that it takes more than three months to recover to the mean preoperative value of 20/25. In our experience, BSCVA after myopic PRK recovers more quickly. We attribute this to the relatively abrupt ablation transition from the untreated central cornea to the corneal margin. (Fig. 6–11) This algorithm represents a considerable departure from the ideal goal of the spherical surface, and this probably leads to multifocal effects in the immediate postoperative period, with impairment of best corrected visual acuity. In our opinion, best corrected visual acuity improves only as a result of subsequent epithelial and stromal changes,

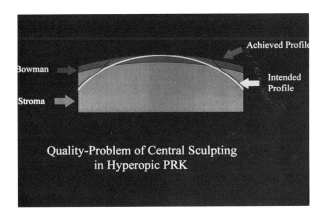

Fig. 6–11. Red line: ablation profile currently used, with abrupt transition from untreated cornea to corneal periphery and deep ablation groove. Due to the multifocal effects caused by this, best-corrected visual acuity recovers only slowly. Yellow line: corneal profile aimed for. This is close to spherical, and leads postoperatively to more rapid recovery of best corrected visual acuity.

with corresponding smoothing of the corneal surface.

Future Plans and Developments

We are attempting to achieve an ablation profile that comes close to a spherical surface by a continuous steepening from the corneal periphery to the central cornea. We assume that best corrected visual acuity will then recover more rapidly than with the present ablation profile and the side effects of halos and night vision disturbances will be reduced.

Predictability

Basing the assessment of predictability on the number of treated eyes within the emmetropic range, i.e., ± 1.00 D, predictability was 81% after 12 months.

Efficacy

The goal of refractive surgery is to improve the patient's uncorrected visual acuity. Hence uncorrected visual acuity is a measure of the efficacy of PRK in this study. Uncorrected visual acuity was 20/40 or better in 66 of 68 eyes (97%).

Stability

Although a 12-month follow-up period may not be long enough for a final analysis of stability, it is sufficient to assess the effectiveness of this method. Ideally, the mean initial correction should be in the minus range. As a result of regression the spherical equivalent regressed from -0.63 ± 1.00 D after one month to $+0.45 \pm 1.16$ D after 12 months (one year regression: 1.08 D). Stability of the spherical equivalent was achieved after six months.

Thereafter there was no statistically significant regression of the correction result. The mean one-year regression was 1.08 D. Of a total of 68 eyes, 62 had a one-year regression of less than 3.00 D, four had a one-year regression of 3.00 D and only one had a regression of 5.00 D. High regressions, up to the preoperative value, were initially reported by many users following treatment with a 7-mm zone, but occurred in our study only in one eye. This observation is in agreement with the results of Kalski et al.,[4] and others who achieved greater stability in myopic PRK with an enlarged treatment zone.[5,6]

Also with the use of a 9-mm treatment zone individuals with high regression up to preoperative values cannot be ruled out, as in myopic-PRK, particularly in eyes with severe decentrations of the treatment zone or dense haze. In the latter case the narrow annular ablation zone is filled completely, with total regression of the correction achieved. To prevent such dense haze formation from the outset, we always use topical steroids.

As reported above, the change in (manual) keratometer readings was significantly less marked than the change in the manifest refractions, and was of only limited value for predicting refraction. Also, in some cases the autorefractor readings showed persistent hyperopia although the manifest refraction did not. This underestimation of the change in refraction is mainly due to the fact that both techniques measure corneal refractive properties at the border of the treated zone.

Alternative methods of H-PRK are hexagonal keratotomy,[7] automated lamellar keratotomy,[8] clear lensectomy with implantation of an intraocular lens (IOL), and holmium laser thermokeratoplasty.[9] Hexagonal keratotomy, automated lamellar keratotomy and clear lensectomy have the disadvantages associated with an invasive procedure. By contrast, PRK is a noncontact procedure. Holmium:YAG laser thermokeratoplasty is not an invasive procedure, however, it is currently recommended only for treating hyperopia up to +4.00 D. Excimer laser PRK can also be used to treat higher hyperopia, up to 8.00 D. Due to the shortage of available literature, a comparative assessment of hyperopic PRK and these alternative procedures is difficult. Only further careful clinical investigations will determine which of these approaches will prevail or the extent to which they will play a dominant role in the correction of hyperopia.

On the basis of the data presented in this paper it may be argued that PRK is an encouraging modality for correcting hyperopia. Evaluation of more cases by more investigators and with longer follow-up should establish the long-term safety and stability of H-PRK. However, it should be mentioned that the results achieved with this method were obtained using the scanning procedure and are not necessarily transferable to other lasers, in particular systems with large-area ablation.

SUMMARY

A prospective clinical study is presented, based on the results of H-PRK in 68 hyperopic eyes (62 patients) using the MEL 60 (Aesculap Meditec) and a 9-mm ablation zone. The mean attempted correction was +4.85 ± 1.45 D (range, +2.00 to +8.25). The maximum follow-up period was 12 months (68 eyes).

Fifty-five eyes (81%) were within ± 1.00 D, 40 eyes (59%) within ± 0.50 D of the intended correction (baseline, +2.00 to +8.25 D) after one year. At 12 months, BCVAs was unchanged or improved in 62 eyes (92%) (safety). Four eyes (6%) had lost one line, one eye (1%) had lost two lines and one eye (1%) three lines. After one year, 66 eyes 97.00% of the eyes had a visual acuity of 20/40 or better (efficacy), 27 eyes (40%) had a visual acuity of 20/40 or better (efficacy).

H-PRK with a 9-mm treatment zone is an efficient and relatively safe procedure for correcting hyperopia of up to +8.25 D. the predictability is good. As in other refractive surgical procedures, great care must be taken to improve the centration of the optical zone.

REFERENCES

1. Dausch D, Klein R, Schroder E: Excimer Laser Photorefractive Keratectomy for Hyperopia. *Refract Corneal Surg* 9:20–28, 1993.
2. Dausch D, Landesz M. Laser correction of hyperopia: Aesculap-Meditec results from German. In Salz JJ, McDonald M, McDonnell PJ, eds.: *Corneal Laser Surgery.* Philadelphia, Pa: Mosby; 1994:pp 237–247.
3. O'Brart DPS, Corbett MC, Verma S, Heacock G, Oliver KM, Lohmann CP, Kerr Muir MG, Marshall J: Effects of Ablation Diameter, Depth, and Edge Contour on the Outcome of Photorefractive Keratectomy. *J Refract Surg* 12:50–60, 1996.
4. Kalski RS, Sutton G, Bin Y, Lawless MA, Rogers C: Comparison of 5-mm and 6-mm Ablation Zones in Photorefractive Keratectomy for Myopia. *J Refract Surg* 12:61–67, 1996.
5. Dausch D, Klein JR, Schroder E: Ophthalmic Excimer Laser Surgery—Clinical Results. *Editions De Signe;* 1991:89–119, 101, 114, 119–126.

6. Ditzen K, Anschutz T, Schroder E: Photorefractive Keratectomy to treat low, medium and high myopia: A multicenter study. *J Cataract Refract Surg. Suppl* 20: 234–238, 1994.

7. Grandon SC, Sanders DR, Anello RD, Jacobs D, Biscaro M: Clinical evaluation of hexagonal keratotomy for the treatment of primary hyperopia. *J Cataract Refract Surg* 21:140–149, 1995.

8. Kezirian GM, Gremillion CM: Automated lamellar keratoplasty for the correction of hyperopia. *J Cataract Refract Surg* 21:386–392, 1995.

9. Yanoff M: Holmium Laser Hyperopia Thermokeratoplasty Update. *Eur J Implant Ref Surg* 7:89–91, 1995.

CHAPTER 7

Presbyopic PRK

Till Anschutz

INTRODUCTION

The surgical correction of presbyopia is a fundamental and an universal challenge. Each year, approximately 51 million people become presbyopic according demographic estimations. In North America alone that number will reach 4 million; in Europe new presbyopes will reach 10 million. This figure is expected to increase considerably as we approach the year 2000.

Etiology of Presbyopia

Rather than an illness, presbyopia seems to be a "feature of senescence: "the progressive loss of accommodation and near visual acuity with age. From 40 to 60 years these symptoms become evident due to aging changes in the lens. However the emergence of this disorder does not depend solely on age. Different factors can have a certain influence. Geographical location with high ultraviolet radiation, accommodative history with high frequency and duration of accommodation and also hypermetropic refractive error can accelerate presbyopia. Myopic people feel this presbyopic effect later than those suffering from hypermetropia. Trauma, drugs, malnutrition, diseases and iatrogenic factors through refractive surgery can also contribute to early presbyopic symptoms. Clear lens extraction, PRK overcorrection, post-RK hyperopic shift after myopic RK and PRK of older patient lead to an untimely onset of presbyopia.

Treatment options have been optical compensation with reading glasses or bifocal and progressive multifocal contact lenses. Halting or prevention of presbyopia is not currently possible, even though researchers continue to investigate potential approaches.[1]

Surgical treatment concepts and methods for presbyopic refractive surgery, which we developed, are relatively new.

Historical Surgical Treatments

The surgical treatment of presbyopia includes different approaches depending on the onset of presbyopia. The refractive surgical treatment of symptomatic presbyopia needs another concept as the iatrogenic presbyopic shift after myopic PRK. The active management to avoid these disadvantages of myopic PRK with loss of near visual acuity in presbyopic myopic patients must lead to a concept to conserve residual myopia through bifocal or multifocal sculpting of the cornea with PRK. This seemed the safest and simplest approach for presbyopia treatment.

MYOPIC-PRESBYOPIC PRK

Observations of unintentional increases of near visual acuity after radial keratotomy[2] and keratomileusis[3], after early postoperative phases of myopic or hyperopic PRK and through corneal scars exhibited as variations in corneal power explain the multifocal lens effect through increased focus depth and positive spherical aberration.[4] This unintentionally created multifocal lens effect produces symptoms of visual distortion or monocular diplopia.[5]

To reproduce these multifocal effects with intentionally calculated corneal power zones we developed a theoretical model of near visual acuity of presbyopic myopic patients through a combined myopia/presbyopia treatment with the excimer laser. We first presented this model September 1990 at the European Excimer Laser congress in Strasbourg.[6,7] Results from our first two patients were presented at the Third International Congress on laser Technology and Ophthalmology in San Francisco in May 1991[8] and at the American Society of Cataract and Refractive Surgery annual meeting in Seattle 1993.[9]

The potential and accuracy of the excimer laser enabled us to create a defined bifocal or multifocal surface of the human cornea similar to the principles of multifocal intraocular lenses (IOL) or contact lenses.[10,11] Disadvantages of unstable focusing through distorted IOLs or bifocal contact lenses do not occur. Trials with various templates (Fig. 7–1) on PMMA lenses and porcine eyes showed the possibility of sculpting multifocal corneas with the excimer laser. The Material Testing Institute of Daimler Benz (Gaggenau, Germany) used high magnification of videomicrography and scanning electron microscopy to show that the treated surfaces have smooth edges of the sectorial zone.

Near Zones

We distinguished two kind of near zones: a central near zone with a peripheral distant zone and a peripheral concentric near zone with a central distant zone (Fig. 7–2.) After experiments with a model eye, and an infra-red laser beam to simulate near rays we developed a third near zone: a sector near zone (Fig. 7–2). The sectorial zone represented part of a concentric zone but was 2 mm within the central zone (Fig. 7–3). The area covered about 2.0 mm^2, sufficient for near vision because the energy received by the retina is proportional to pupil size.[12] This sector zone had, we believe, some advantages. The simple concentric multifocal zone[13] is not ideal for the human cornea because it does not provide smooth transition zones. Dependent on pupil size these zones diminish the dis-

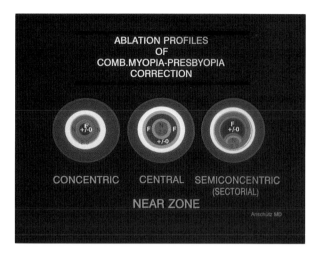

Fig. 7–2. Ablation concepts of combined myopia-presbyopia correction with different near zones.

tant central zone. Areas smaller than 1.4 mm^2 limit visual acuity to less than 20/20.[14] A small distant central zone of 1.5 mm and an additional transition zone of nearly 0.5 mm implies a minimal pupil diameter of 4 mm. The known effect of aging in reducing pupil size[15,16] causes small pupils and progressive regression of the distance zone with increasing loss of distance acuity and more glare, halo and scatter effects through the larger border area of the concentric zone.[17] We abandoned this concentric multifocal concept because of the high dependency on larger pupil size for optimal performance.[18] Koch and colleagues have shown that mean pupil size at a reading illumination of 80 (ft-c registered by lightmeter) is 2.8 mm for patients 40 to 59 years old.[14]

Pseudoaccommodation

The effect of bifocal or multifocal IOLs or contact lenses is based on the reception of simultaneous images at the retina through various foci.[19,20,21] The ability to process these different images is called pseudoaccommodation. Physiological aspects of vision and the interaction of multifocal imagery have not been fully investigated, although some reports seem to confirm the benefit of a bifocal system.[22] The human retina recognizes only one image; parallel perception is not possible. An important factor of multifocal vision is the individual ability of pseudoaccommodation and the capability of the multifocal cornea to produce comfortable vision. We describe these abilities of increased depth of

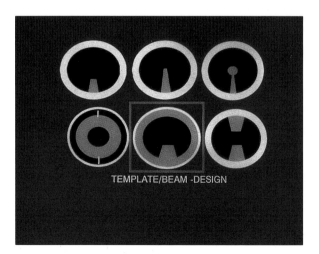

Fig. 7–1. Various templates for sculpting multifocal cornea.

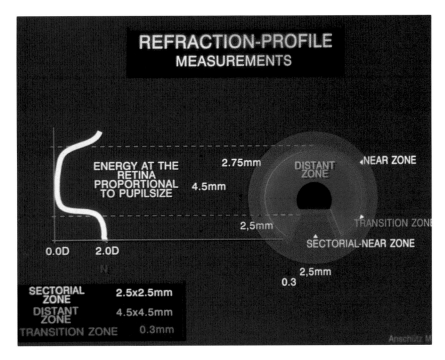

Fig. 7–3. Corneal refractive power and ablation measurements after myopic-presbyopic PRK.

focus and the perception of a focal interval as "polymetropia" (Fig. 7–5).

Types of Pseudoaccommodation

There are two types of pseudoaccommodation: near dominance and distant dominance. We investigated a peripheral/sectorial near zone concept with pupil size dependence and far visual dominance; a central near zone concept less dependent on pupil size and near visual dominance (Fig. 7–2) was also studied. The ray model demonstrates this situation after monofocal myopic PRK. The distant rays were focused on the retina, the near rays were focused behind the retina. After multifocal myopic/presbyopic PRK, the expected focus of the near rays is also on the retina through the less ablated sectorial or central near zone (Fig. 7–4). This method should improve the disadvantages of monofocal myopic

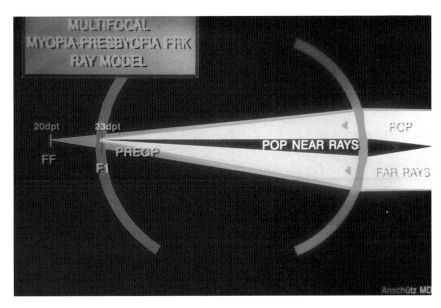

Fig. 7–4. Ray model of multifocal myopic-presbyopic PRK pre- and post-operative.

PRK with loss of near visual acuity. Our multifocal myopia/presbyopia study began in March 1991; to date 560 patients have been treated.

The avoidance of presbyopic shift after myopic PRK by creating different corneal power zones through reduced ablation depth and diminished corneal flattening is a kind of passive myopization, because a defined part of the cornea remains less or untreated corresponding to a spherical equivalent of -2.00 to -3.00 D as residual myopia. The treatment of symptomatic or iatrogenic presbyopia requires a method for active myopization through steepening the cornea to create a positive sphericity. We noticed that in the early postoperative phases of hyperopic PRK the near visual acuity also increased. This effect disappeared after several weeks. Similar to the sectorial passive myopization of the combined myopia/presbyopia treatment we wanted to create a positive asphericity through partial steepening of the cornea. The theoretical basis was the Gaussian system of cardinal points in the Gullstrand schematic eye[23] and JB Listing[24] who was the first to propose that the eye be considered in such a simple fashion. Sturm's conoid (Fig. 7–5) illustrates the understanding of the physical aspect of varying corneal curvatures.

The simulation of these reflections through experimental treatment of PMMA contact lenses with the excimer laser and ablating of the inferior part of cornea epithelium preceded the following study. Similar effects showed the impression of the peripheral cornea with the Sinskey Hook. This partial corneal steepening significantly improved the near visual acuity through progression of the corneal curvature with increasing deflection of the near ray traces (Fig. 7–6).

To reach this goal we attempted a partial steepening through a defined sectorial hyperopic ablation with an asymmetric positive aspheric curvature (Fig. 7–7). The initial treatments combined the hyperopic rotation spiral template; in later applications the new hyperopic "double-heart rotating template" (Fig. 7–8) with a nonrotating presbyopic template and an oval opening was used.

After encouraging results with the sectorial corneal profiling to steepen a defined part of the cornea to create a convex optical system, we developed a special presbyopic rotating template (Fig. 7-9) to treat simple presbyopia.

This emmetropia/hyperopia/presbyopia study began in July 1992 with 20 cases. The theoretical model was first presented in September 1992[7,25] and initial results of treated cases appeared in 1993.[7,26]

Fig. 7–5. Sturm's conoid: Illustration of the bundle of rays at different points at *A*. A section of the bundle will be in the form of a horizontal oval ellipse. At *B*, the vertical rays come to a focus, whereas the horizontal rays are still converting (horizontal straight line). Beyond B, the vertical rays diverge whereas the horizontal are still converging. At first at *C*, the bundle will be a horizontal oval ellipse. At *D* the section becomes a circle. The least amount of distortion takes place here. This is called the *circle of least confusion*. Beyond this point, the divergence of the vertical rays dominates, and an ellipse again is formed. (*E*). The horizontal rays up to *F* come to a focus; beyond *G*, both sets of rays are always diverging. The section will take the form of a gradually increasing vertical oval.

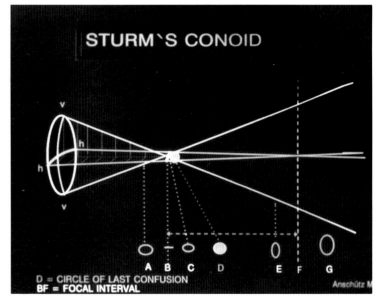

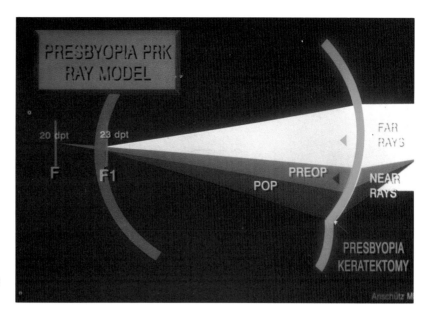

Fig. 7–6. Ray model of simple presbyopic PRK pre- and postoperatively.

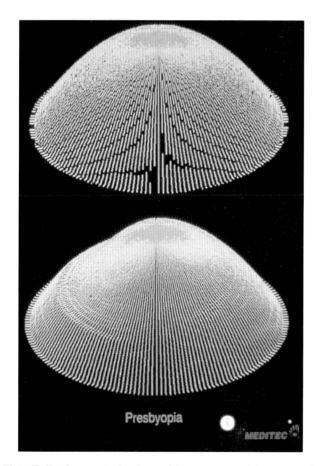

Fig. 7–7. Computerized positive asymmetric corneal asphericity.

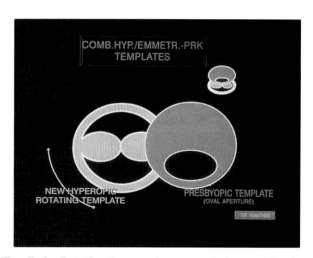

Fig. 7–8. Rotating hyperopic eyemask in combination with presbyopic template.

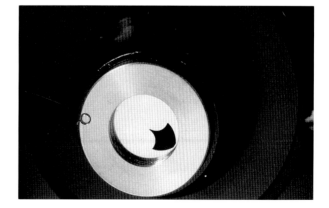

Fig. 7–9. Presbyopic rotating hand-hold eyemask with spearlike aperture.

CURRENT SURGICAL TECHNIQUE

Examination of pseudoaccommodation with multi-focal lenses (Variation™ Lunelle) was attempted, but not always helpful. Unstable focusing due to floating contact lenses sometimes simulated pseu-doaccommodation problems. The stability of fixed multifocal zones after multifocal PRK may be an advantage compared to multifocal contact lenses.

A preoperative explanation of the risks of regression, visual disturbances, under- or overcorrection was given to each patient. Preliminary discussions and detailed printed information explained possible postoperative complications such as glare, haze, scars, diplopia, and steroid response leading to a rise in intraocular pressure.

Patients understood the investigational nature of the treatment; each patient gave written consent prior to surgery. Cycloplegic and manifest refractions, uncorrected and best corrected visual acuity, slit-lamp and fundus examination, videokeratos-copy, biometry, pachymetry, tonometry, contrast sensitivity, and a defocus test were given pre- and postoperatively. Trials with multifocal and bifocal contact lenses were always performed. Postoperative care and regimen were identical to that for hyperopic or myopic PRK. Patient exams were performed on postoperative days one, two, three and during months one, three, six, nine, twelve, twenty-four, thirty-six and forty-eight. All treated eyes were fitted with soft disposable bandage lenses (Acuvue™, NuVue™) immediately postoperatively for two days. Antibiotic drugs and protective gels (Actovegin®) were given for 10 days with additional application of topical heparin.[26,27] After re-epithelialization, usually 10 days postoperative, fluorometholone 0.1% was prescribed for six months.

The ablation depth for +2.00 D of additional presbyopia was 20 μm; for an intended presbyopic correction of +3.00 D, ablation was 30 μm deeper. The ray model (Fig. 7–6) shows pre- and postpres-byopic PRK. The distance rays have been focused on the retina, the near rays behind the retina. After presbyopic or hyperopic/presbyopic PRK the expected focus of near rays was also on the retina through the additional steepening of the cornea curvature. The cross-section ablation profile of a combined hyperopic/presbyopic PRK is shown in Fig. 7–10A, the cross-section ablation profile of the emmetropic/presbyopic PRK is shown in Fig. 7–10B.

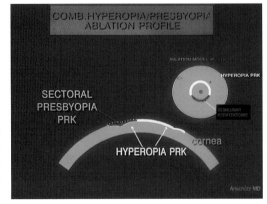

Fig. 7–10A. Cross-section of a combined hyperopia-presbyopia PRK with the profile of simple hyperopic and additionally presby-opic sectorial keratectomy.

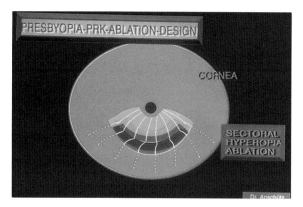

Fig. 7–10B. Cross-section of a simple presbyopic keratectomy.

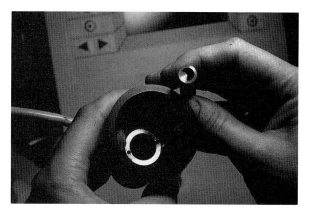

Fig. 7–11. Combination of a hand-hold iris diaphragm for myopic PRK and nonrotating sectorial template for creating sectorial near zone.

SURGICAL TECHNIQUE

A 193 nm excimer laser (MEL 60 Aesculap Meditec, Heroldsberg, Germany) with a suction ring and hand-held diaphragm was used. The aim was to create discrete refraction zones by sculpting the cornea. Preoperative surgical management was similar to that for myopic or hyperopic PRK: topical anesthesia with proparacaine; insertion of the eyelid speculum; patient self-fixation in the operating microscope light; marking of the visual axis with a Sinskey hook; marking of the ablation zone with a radial keratotomy optical zone marker; and epithelial debridement with the hockey knife. After carefully cleaning the central debridement area of any cellular debris, the suction ring with the hand-held mask is placed on the eye. The risk of a decentered ablation with resultant irregular astigmatism and unpredictable outcomes is diminished through this intraoperatively active eye fixation by the surgeon. Postoperatively, the treated area was immediately rinsed with balanced saline solution (BSS). The ablation zone was covered with Healon® and a therapeutic bandage lens.

Combined Myopic/Presbyopic PRK

An iris diaphragm for myopic PRK was used for the myopic/presbyopic treatment. The ablation was dependent on the age of the patient; usually 2 to 3 D less than the myopic baseline refraction. In the second phase, a sectorial template based on a cylindrical hand-holder in the iris diaphragm (eyemask with suction ring, Fig. 7–11) was inserted to fixate the globe during ablation. For the central near zone, a nonrotating modified template was used. An example of the treatment steps for a presbyopic/ myopic patient with a −5.00 D refraction and an additional intended presbyopic correction of +2.00 D demonstrates this method. To correct −1.00 D, an ablation depth of nearly 9 μm is needed. For this reason, the first ablation is 18 μm deep, corresponding to a value of −2.00 D and an uncorrected residual value of 3.00 D. After inserting the special sectorial or central template in the maskholder, a second ablation of 27 μm corresponding to the residual noncorrected value of −3.00 D was performed. With these two ablations an average ablation depth of 45 μm was achieved, corresponding to the baseline refraction of −5.00 D (Fig. 7–12A). By partially protecting the first treated ablation zone with the sectorial or central presbyopic templates we created a sectorial or central near zone with an expected residual value of −2.00 D and a distance zone with an expected plano (Fig. 7–12B,C).

Hyperopic/Presbyopic PRK

The main technical requirement for hyperopic/presbyopic PRK was a rotating mask for hyperopic sculpting of the cornea (Fig. 7–8) with a suction ring. In the first ablation phase hyperopic PRK corresponding to the hyperopic baseline of refraction was performed with a rotating mask. In the second phase a nonrotating presbyopic template with an oval aperture mounted on a metal cylinder in the hyperopic eye mask holder (Fig. 7–8) was inserted. The position selected allowed an additional sectorial

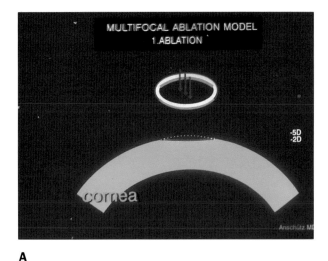

A

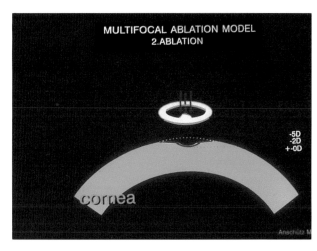

B

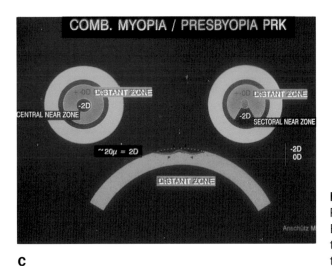

C

Fig. 7–12. Ablation process of two step myopic-presbyopic PRK: A. myopic ablation phase with myopic iris diaphragm, B. additional myopic ablation in combination with the protecting sectorial/central near zone templates, C. cross-section of the postoperative ablation profile.

inferior hyperopic ablation. Because of the design we called this kind of ablation semilunar keratectomy (SLK). The additional ablation depth in this treatment were 20 μm, corresponding to +2.00 D of intended presbyopic correction, and nearly 30 μm, corresponding to +3.00 D (Fig. 10A).

Emmetropic/Presbyopic PRK

The same hyperopic masks described above were used in emmetropic/presbyopic PRK with the oval template (Fig. 7–8) to create a defined inferiorly steepened corneal ablation profile (Fig. 7–7). To achieve an aspherical steepening for an intended presbyopic correction of 3.00 D, we ablated a sec-

torial zone of 30 μm depth (Fig. 7–10B). To achieve a smoother transition zone we combined this with a concentric steepening of 0.50 D. The semilunar-like ablation angle was 60°. The development of a rotating presbyopic hand-held mask with a spear-like aperture and suction ring (Fig. 7–9) simplified this technique. With a special computerized program developed by S. Pieger[7] it was possible to sculpt a defined partial aspherical steepening of the cornea. The rotation speed with small angle steps is slower in the 60-degree sectorial zone, and faster, with larger angle steps, in the transition zone.

These altered angle distances allow the creation of different ablation depths during the rotation in the desired sectorial zone and in the untreated zone to

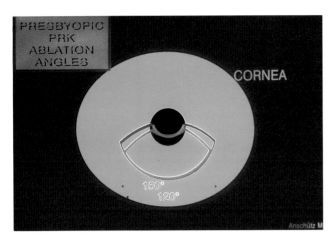

Fig. 7–13. Various ablation angles for sculpting semilunar like corneal steepening with the rotating presbyopic mask.

reach a smooth and softer transition.[7] This system also allows various ablation angles between 80° and 150° (Fig. 7–13) and the creation of semilunar, positive asymmetric asphericity in different parts of the cornea.

CLINICAL RESULTS

Multifocal Myopic/Presbyopic PRK

Our multifocal myopic/presbyopic PRK study that we began April 1991 has a five-year follow-up.

patients have a significant improvement in uncorrected near visual acuity.[7]

Group I comprised of 31 eyes with refraction ranging from −2.00 to −6.00 D. Group II had refractions ranging from −6.50 to −10.00 D. Ages ranged from 45 to 64 years, with a mean age of 54 years. The intended presbyopic correction was 2.00 to 3.00 D. Twenty-four eyes in group I had regression similar to that observed after monofocal ablation. The immediate postoperative overcorrection averaged +1.50 D and regressed over time to a mean of −1.50 D (Fig. 7–14). The uncorrected visual acuity (UCVA) had slight regression to a near visual acuity of J3. A comparative monofocal-treated group had a loss 1.5 lines UCVA.

Causes for Loss of Near Visual Acuity

Causes for the decrease of near visual acuity are additional age-related loss of near visual acuity and epithelialization of the near zone. In the monofocal group, an improved near visual acuity one year postoperative is seen, depending on myopic regression. Over five years, however, these eyes also had a loss of near visual acuity due to aging.

In Group II (−6.50 to −10.00 D) similar effects were seen. The higher regression, up to −4.00 D, helped to balance the difference between multifocally and monofocally treated eyes. The higher regression in Group II led to diminished distance vision without correction and to consequent enhancement of near visual acuity. The comparison

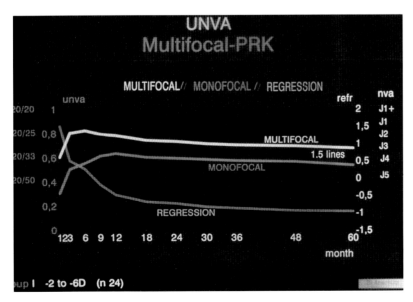

Fig. 7–14. Multifocal myopia-presbyopia. Comparison monofocal/multifocal PRK concerning near visual acuity.

of monofocally and multifocally treated eyes with the defocus test (Fig. 7–15) showed a significantly better near acuity of the multifocally treated eyes. Haze density varied in different refraction zones. The less ablated near zone was clearer. The borderline of the near refraction zones occasionally developed brown pigment lines. We found only a small loss of contrast sensitivity in the group of sectorial near-zone treated patients.

Group III consisted of six eyes, those with preoperative refractions from −10.00 to −15.00 D. These eyes had improved UCVA. Because of near dominant pseudoaccommodation of highly myopic patients, we treated them with the central near zone option. Uncorrected near visual acuity was improved in the first year, although there was significant regression to a mean of −6.70 D.

Videokeratography (Fig. 7–16) shows the different ablation zones. The superficial multifocal effect disappears over time in many cases. Near visual acuity with full distance correction was 1.6 lines better than near visual acuity in the monofocal-treated group.

With the laser interferometer (Class™ 1000) it was possible to demonstrate differences on the remaining multifocal refraction zones. The objective refractometry of multifocal zones with currently available refractometers is not possible. A potential measurement method is the infrared retinoscope (Viva™ Tomey, Germany). Fifty-four percent of eyes developed higher halo and glare effects in the first six postoperative months than that seen in monofocally treated eyes. After six months these effects decreased in most cases. The spread of light distribution as indicators of vision was not very marked in the point spread function.

Visual Disturbances

There was a problem in adapting to two foci. After approximately four weeks, the brain adapted to the multifocal images, although 20% of patients complained for three or four months about ghosting and diplopia. These visual disturbances disappeared over time. In cases with central near zones the complaints about monocular diplopia were significantly more frequent. Patients with small pupils ($\geq$ 2 mm) had worse uncorrected distance visual acuity. In four cases the near zone was too large with residual distance visual problems. In three cases the pupil size was smaller than 2 mm with reduced uncorrected near visual acuity. It is our clinical impression that visual recovery is two to three weeks longer in these eyes compared to monofocal myopic

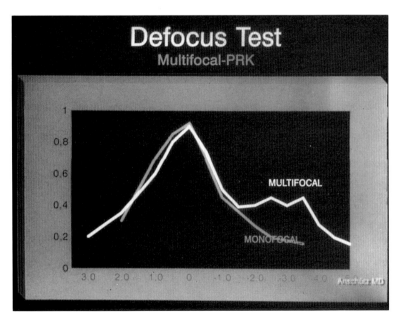

Fig. 7–15. Defocus-test. Comparison of monofocal and multifocal ablation.

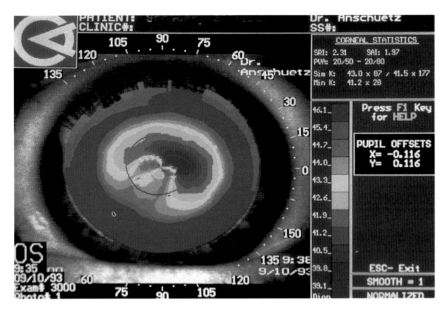

Fig. 7–16. Videokeratoscopy of different refraction zones after multifocal myopia/presbyopia PRK with sectorial near zone.

treated eyes. One eye of 23 eyes lost two lines of BCVA from decentration.

Simple Presbyopic and Hyperopic/Presbyopic PRK

Our presbyopia study started in July 1992 with 20 cases. Ages ranged between 48 and 63 years, with a preoperative baseline refraction from plano to +8.00 D. These patients were divided into three groups: group Ia (plano to +0.50 D), group Ib, (+1.00 to +4.75 D); and group II, +5.00 to +8.00 D. After a follow-up of three years, group Ib had a mean regression of nearly +1.80 D and a mean UCVA of J4 at a reading distance of 37cm. Group II developed significantly higher regression of +4.20 D with a much lower near visual acuity of J8 (Fig. 7–17A and 7–17B).

The best results were seen in the emmetropic/presbyopic group with an enhancement of UCVA of 2.3 lines over 36 months. The infrared retinoscopy provided a helpful way to measure objectively the presbyopic effect visible on videokeratoscopy (Fig. 7–18). Presbyopic PRK affected distance visual acuity with a myopic cylindric shift (−0.25 to −1.00 D) in the first three postoperative months. Reduced distance visual acuity and an improved uncorrected visual acuity were observed.

After three months, distance visual acuity returned to preoperative levels. In this emmetropic,

simple presbyopic group, no eye lost more than two lines. The main problem was that 50% of patients complained of ghosting and diplopia, which disappeared by six months postoperatively. In 5% of the cases the effect remained. The causes for this problem could be the appearance of a bundle of rays at different points; the known adapting phase of pseudoaccommodation; and slight iatrogenic irregular astigmatism. Interestingly the least problems with ghosting occurred in those 45 to 55 years of age.

Changing of the asymmetric positive asphericity from the inferior to the upper cornea has no significant influence concerning near visual acuity. This leads us to the suggestion that the capability of pseudoaccommodation is a complex learning process related to age and intelligence. Most patients over 60 years had obvious problems in processing multifocal images.

Further Studies

First year data of the European multicenter study from Smecka et al. (personal communication, 1995) seem to confirm the above considerations. From the end of 1994, the group evaluated 35 eyes (initial correction −0.25 D to +0.50 D). The postoperative regimen was identical to that previously described. FML was applied only once or twice a day, according to the postoperative results. At the beginning was the nondominant eye operated. In most cases,

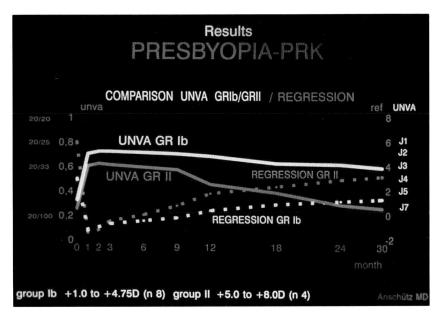

A

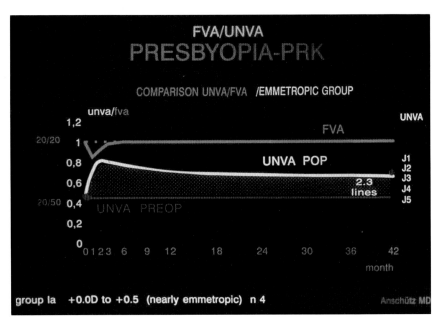

Fig. 7–17. Regression after PRK and uncorrected visual acuity.

B

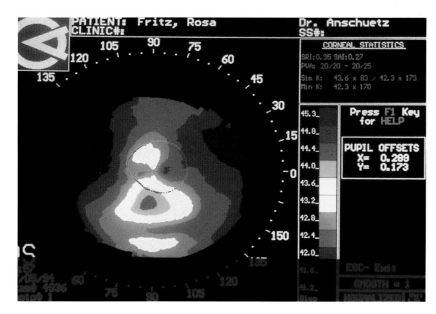

Fig. 7–18. Videokeratoscopy of simple presbyopic PRK with typical inferior steepening.

PRK was performed in the upper half of the cornea. Visual perception for near distance adjusted very soon.

Alteration in far visual acuity was seen in the first two months and increased almost regularly. The usual postoperative values of refraction for distance adjusts to plano to −0.50 spherical and −0.5 to −1.25 cylindrical usually in axis 180°. Correction for the near distance was very stable with +0.25 D from the planned correction, only one regression of 0.75 D was seen.

DISCUSSION

After nearly more than 560 myopic/presbyopic cases treated with this technique, we believe that this method may be a viable option in treating presbyopic shift after myopic PRK of presbyopic patients and in improving UCVA. The complication rate is similar to that for monofocal-treated eyes. However, the procedure is dependent on near/far dominance, pupil size. There is a considerable risk of scatter and halo effects. Ghosting, reduced far visual acuity and regression remain considerable effects that must be assessed. An alternative treatment to compensate for presbyopic shift after

myopic PRK is monovision. Risks include aniseikonia and late anisometropia of more than 1.50 D. We abandoned unilateral PRK in favor of multifocal myopic/presbyopic treatment. Fig. 7-19 shows several ablation profiles depending on the preoperative situation. Myopic/presbyopic treatments with a central near zone are no longer done due to a higher incidence of monocular diplopia and the loss of distance visual acuity. Central islands may provide similar visual symptoms.

This treatment requires careful patient selection. The processing of multifocal images with the alternate suppression of far and near foci seems to be an intellectual learning process and needs certain intellectual abilities. Tests to exclude the inability of pseudoaccommodation may be helpful in improving treatment success. Relation to age and intelligence are important; patients over 60 years old are now treated only in selected cases. This is similar to problems noted with multifocal IOLs. Fig. 7-20 shows the relationship to with age and satisfaction. As the patients increased in age, the satisfaction decreased.

After 110 simple presbyopic PRKs we believe in the following options for presbyopic PRK. The preliminary results are encouraging, but challenging. To date primary presbyopia therapy is not standard-

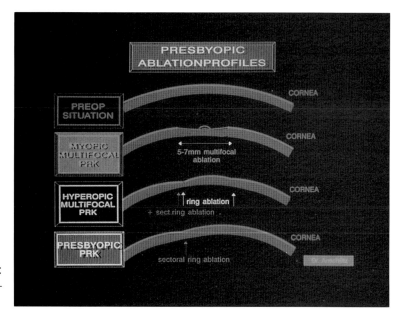

Fig. 7–19. Various presbyopic PRK—profiles: myopic-, hyperopic- and emmetropic—presbyopic PRK.

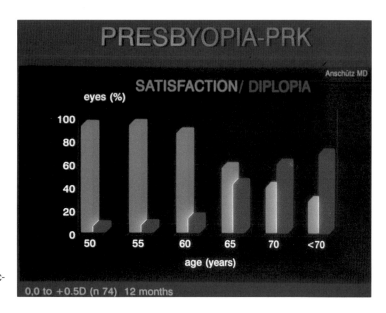

Fig. 7–20. Age relation dependence to satisfaction diplopia.

ized. Results of a multicenter study at 10 sites in Europe are encouraging. In the future, it is imperative that we have a better understanding of the interaction of multifocal images and the cerebral compensation for defects in the human optical system. Possible refinements through new aspheric cornea curvature designs would be beneficial.

REFERENCES

1. Pierscionek B, Weale RA: Symposium International de la Presbytie June 5–9, 1995, France.
2. Santos VR, Waring GO III, Lynn MJ, Holladay JT, Sperduto RD: PERK Study Group. Relationship between refractive error and visual acuity in the

Prospective Evaluation of Radial Keratotomy (PERK) Study. *Arch Ophthalmol* 105:86–92, 1987.

3. Moreira H, Garbus JJ, Lee M, et al. Multifocal corneal topographic changes after radial keratotomy, *Arch Ophthalmol* 110:994–999, 1992.

4. Holladay JT, Lynn MJ, Waring GO III, Gemmilli M, Keehn GC, Fielding B: The relationship of visual acuity, refractive error, and pupil size after radial keratotomy. *Arch Ophthalmol* 90: 70–76, 1991.

5. Maguire LJ, Bourne WM: A multifocal lens effect as a complication of radial keratotomy. *Refract Corneal Surg* 6:394–397, 1989.

6. Anschütz T: Theoretic model of a combined presbyopia PRK. Presented at the European Excimer Laser Congress, 1990, Strasbourg, France.

7. Anschütz T: Laser correction of hyperopia and presbyopia. *Int Ophthal Clin* 34:105–135, 1994.

8. Anschütz T: Model of a combined presbyopia correction with the excimer-laser and report of treated cases. Presented at the Third International Congress on Laser Technology in Ophthalmology, 1991, San Francisco, CA.

9. Anschütz T: Multifocal excimer PRK combined myopia-presbyopia treatment. American Society of Cataract and Refractive Surgery, May 93, Seattle, Washington abstracts p. 104.

10. Holladay JT, Dijk Hvan, Lang A, et al: Optical performance of multifocal intraocular lenses. *J Cataract Refract Surg* 16:413–422, 1990.

11. Maxwell WA: Introduction to the current status of multifocal intraocular lenses. In Maxwell WA, Nordan LT, eds: *Current Concepts of Multifocal Intraocular Lenses.* Thorofare, NJ: Slack. 1991, 3–11.

12. Duke-Elder S: *The Pupil. Textbook of Ophthalmology.* St. Louis, Mosby, 1954, p 555.

13. Krüger RR, McDonnell PJ: New directions in excimer-laser surgery. In Thompson FB, McDonnell PJ, ed: *Excimer Laser Surgery,* Tokyo: Igaku-Schoin, 1993, pp 143–144.

14. Koch DD, Samuelson SW, Hatt EA: Merin LM. Pupillary responsiveness and its implications for selection of a bifocal intraocular lens. In Maxwell WA, Nordan LT, eds: *Current Concepts of Multifocal Intraocular Lenses.* Thorofare. NJ: Slack. 1991, 147–152.

15. Loewenfeld JE: Pupillary changes related to age. In Thompson HS, Daroff R, Frisen L, Glaser JS, Sanders MD: *Topics in Neuro-Ophthalmology.* Baltimore USA. Williams and Wilkens, 1973, pp 124–150.

16. Loewenfeld JE: *The Pupil.* Detroit, Wayne State University Press, 1993, pp 295–317.

17. Anschütz T: Pupil size, ablation diameter and halo incidence after Photorefractive Keratectomy. ASCRS Symposium on Cataract, IOL Refract Surg 1995; pp 1–4.

18. Kadlecova V, Peleska M, Vasko A: Dependence on age of the diameter of the pupil in the dark. *Nature* 182:1520–1521, 1958.

19. Knorz MC, Claessens D, Schaefer RC, et al: Evaluation of contrast acuity and defocus curve in bifocal and monofocal IOLs. *J Cataract Refract Surg* 19:513–523, 1993.

20. Knorz MC, Koch DD, Martinez-Franco, C., Lorger CV: Effect of pupil size and astigmatism on contrast acuity with monofocal and bifocal intraocular lenses. *J Cataract Refract Surg* 20:26–33, 1994.

21. Chipman RA: Image formation by multifocal lenses. In Maxwell WA, Nordan LT eds: *Current Concepts of Multifocal Intraocular Lenses.* Thorofare. NJ: Slack; 1991, pp 37–52.

22. Roth EH: Sinnesphysiologische Aspekte des Sehens mit bifokalen intraocular Linsen. *DGII* 266–269, 1992.

23. Gullstrand. Hb d. physiologischen Optik von H. v. Helmholtz, ed 3. Hamburg, 1 (1909) Einführung in d. Methoden d. Dioptrik d. Auges d. Menschen. Leipzig, 1911.

24. Listing JB: Zur Dioptrik d. Auges. In *Wagner's Handwörterbuch der Physiologie* Braunschweig 1853, 4:451.

25. Anschütz T. Theoretic model of simple presbyopia PRK. DELV Symposium, 1992, Mannheim, Germany.

26. Anschütz T, Presbyopia PRK. DOG Der Augenspiegel 40(2):46–48, 1994.

27. Vanns S: Experimental and clinical investigations into the effect of locally administered heparin on the eye. *Acta Ophthalmol Suppl* 49, 1952.

28. Salomaa S: Experiments with heparin. *Acta Ophthalmol.* 30:33, 1952.

29. Baltes P, Lindenberger U: Im Alter schwindet die Intelligenz. *Welt* 8, 1996.

CHAPTER 8

Excimer Laser Photorefractive Keratectomy For Hyperopia (PRK)

Summit Technology's Experience

Michael Lawless

INTRODUCTION

Photorefractive keratectomy (PRK) using the excimer laser is now a well established procedure for the correction of low to moderate degrees of myopia, and more recently, for the correction of myopic astigmatism.[1,2] Excimer laser correction for hyperopia has proved to be more difficult with very little data published in the peer review literature. The problem has not been that hyperopic correction has not been possible, but that the effect has been transitory with regression of refractive effect over time. We began treating hyperopia in June 1995 with the introduction of the Summit SVS Apogee laser (now called the SVS Apex plus) and hyperopic mask in rail technology and Axicon lens.

The principle of treatment for hyperopia with this system is relatively straight forward. The sequence is manual epithelial debridement to allow for a 10 mm zone, treatment with a 6.5 mm zone hyperopic mask of determined power, and then treatment with an Axicon lens to diverge the beam and create a trough between 6.5 and 9.4 mm as an annulus zone.

METHOD

Patients are prepared in the usual manner for PRK with topical local anaesthesia (Amethocaine 1.0%) and one drop of Pilocarpine 2% 20 minutes prior to the procedure. No oral sedative is used preoperatively.

The patient is positioned under the laser and is given practice at fixating on the green, blinking, fixation light. The surgeon assesses patient fixation and cooperation via the operating microscope (aided by two helium neon aiming beams positioned at three and nine o'clock either side of the visual axis). A speculum is inserted and manual debridement of the corneal epithelium is performed using a sterile blunted hockey blade. For hyperopic corrections, since the ablation zone is 9.4 mm, most of the corneal epithelium needs to be removed. We have found that hyperopic eyes tend to have a slightly smaller diameter than normal and myopic eyes. Therefore, occasionally in removing the corneal epithelium, one needs to go quite close to the limbus. It is important to leave a cuff of remaining epithelium. Occasionally bleeding will occur particularly if there has been previous contact lens wear with pannus development in the corneal periphery. Attention needs to be directed to this with all bleeding controlled prior to proceeding.

Once the corneal epithelium is satisfactorily removed, the surface is dried and patient fixation checked once again. At this stage a hyperopic mask is inserted into the down rail of the laser and this can be from 1.0 to 4.0 diopters (in 0.5 diopter steps). With each mask power there are a certain number of pulses to be programmed as outlined in Table 8–1.

The operating microscope light is turned off and patient fixation checked again. The ablation commences beginning at the 6.5 mm zone working towards the visual axis. This creates an ablation profile the reverse of a myopic PRK with very little ablation centrally in the visual axis and most of the ablation occurring in the mid periphery.

The operating light is turned on, the cassette removed from the down rail of the laser and the laser re-programmed for the Axicon portion of the procedure. The Axicon lens diverges the beam to deliver energy between 6.5 mm and 9.4 mm (Fig.

Table 8–1. Hyperopic Algorithm

Diopters	Number of Axicon Shots
+1.00	79
+2.00	177
+3.00	275
+4.00	372

8–1), with the maximum energy delivered at 6.5 mm and the energy delivered tapering off as the beam approaches 9.4 mm (Fig. 8–2). This creates a maximal effect at the 6.5 mm to 7.5 mm zone creating a trough in an attempt to have a blend zone over the treated area of the cornea which will stabilize the central cornea and hopefully limit regression (Fig. 8–3). The Axicon lens is inserted within its own cassette in the down rail of the laser. A schematic is shown in Fig. 8–4. The patient is again asked to fix the fixation light, the corneal surface is dried with a sterile sponge, the surface checked and then the ablation commences. Total time for the procedure tends to be less then five minutes. The time taken for epithelial debridement can be two to three minutes, as a more complete debridement is necessary than with myopic PRK due to the larger ablation zone. The first hyperopic mask ablation takes

approximately 30 seconds and then there is a forty-five second delay for re-programming. The final Axicon ablation takes approximately 30 seconds. At the end of the procedure, Cyclopentolate 1% and an antibiotic are applied and the patient patched. The pressure patch is maintained for thirty-six hours and topical antibiotics are then continued until re-epithelialization occurs. Oral medication for pain (Panadeine Forte) is supplied and a sleeping tablet (Rohypnol 2 mg) is also given to the patient for the first postoperative night. The patient is also given a vial of Minims of Amethocaine 0.5% in case of severe pain (to be used on the first postoperative night if required).

Once re-epithelialization has occurred, generally at day three, topical corticosteroids (Fluoromethalone 0.1%) drops are used twice a day for four weeks.

RESULTS

The results using this technique are preliminary with nine-month data available on a prospective study of 11 hyperopic eyes of 11 patients (ten phakic and one aphakic). These patients underwent excimer laser correction of their hyperopia on 20th June, 1995 at the Sydney Refractive Surgery

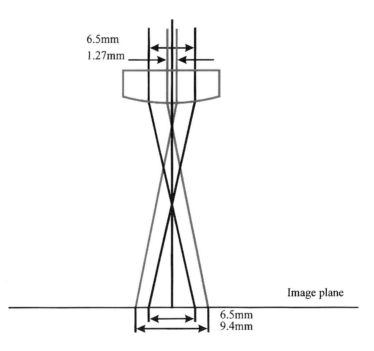

Fig. 8–1. Schematic of laser and axicon lens system

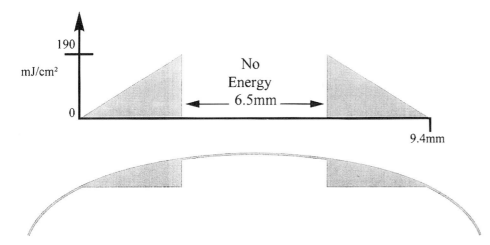

Fig. 8–2. Schematic of axicon lens showing central 6.5 mm and blend zone created by axicon lens to 9.5 mm. This creates a maximal effect at the 6.5 mm to 7.5 mm zone creating a trough in an attempt to have a blend zone over the treated area of the cornea which will stabilize the central cornea and hopefully limit regression

Center. Full informed consent was obtained and approval given by the participating hospital Ethics Committee for this investigational trial. Data included cycloplegic refraction, best spectacle corrected acuity, degree of corneal haze, manual keratometry and computer assisted video topography with the Eyesys topographic unit. The data was collected preoperatively and at predetermined review visits at one, two, three, six and nine months.

Preoperative hyperopic refraction ranged from +2.50 to +8.38 diopters (spherical equivalent) at the spectacle plane. This equated to a mean of +5.90 diopters at the corneal plane. Attempted correction was +2.0, +3.0 or +4.0 diopters at the corneal plane using the combination hyperopic mask followed by an Axicon lens. The mean attempted correction was +3.09 diopters at the corneal plane. Refraction data for the overall group

- Use laser disc for 6.5mm optical correction

- Axicon creates 9.4mm blend zone

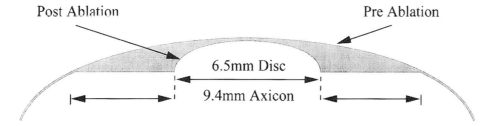

Fig. 8–3. Hyperopic correction with axicon.

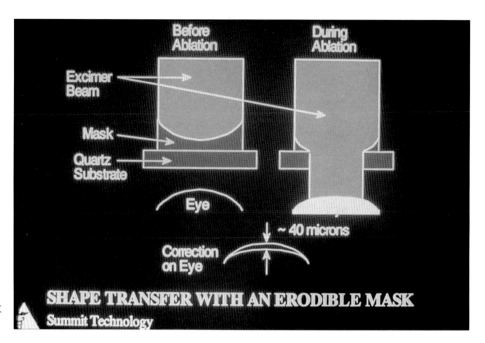

Fig. 8–4. Schematic of Summit Apogee SVS laser system

showed a mean initial overcorrection at four weeks of +3.18 diopters (SD 1.60) that regressed slightly before stabilizing at about twelve weeks with a mean overcorrection of +1.88 diopters (SD 1.03). Thereafter there was no statistically significant fluctuation in refraction. The degree of overcorrection was greater in the higher treatment groups. Similarly the degree of regression was greater in the higher treatment groups. Keratometry results correlated more closely to attempted hyperopic correction. Stabilization of keratometry readings did not occur until twenty-four weeks. Again there was an initial overcorrection. For the group overall, this was a mean overcorrection of +1.83 diopters (SD 1.11) by manual keratometry and +0.90 diopters (SD 0.83) by computer-assisted video topography. By 24 weeks, manual keratometry mean overcorrection was zero (SD 1.56), while on topography, there was a mean undercorrection of 0.64 diopters (SD 1.76). As with refraction, the degree of overcorrection and regression was greater in the higher treatment groups. Corneal haze was limited to the mid peripheral cornea and was visually insignificant. By the ninth month review none of the patients reviewed had suffered any loss in best corrected

visual acuity, and one patient gained one line in best corrected spectacle visual acuity. If we look at the data in more detail, we see that 3 patients underwent a 2 diopter hyperopic correction, 3 patients a 3 diopter, and 4 patients a 4 diopter hyperopic correction.

The refraction data for the group as a whole showed that at four weeks, the mean refraction was a spherical equivalent of −0.49 diopters (SD 0.85) at the glasses plane that equated to a mean overcorrection of +3.18 diopters (SD 1.6). Table 8–2 reveals that there was some regression over eight weeks with refraction stabilizing at about twelve weeks to a spherical equivalent of +1.04 diopters (SD 0.8) at the glasses plane, equating to a mean overcorrection of +1.92 diopters (SD 1.15). Tables 8–3 to 8–5 reveal the mean correction for individual groups of 2.0, 3.0 and 4.0 diopter masks. The 2 diopter treatment group showed only very slight regression from an initial mean overcorrection of +1.68 diopters (SD 0.21) at four weeks to +1.52 diopters (SD 0.6) at 24 weeks. There was an increase in the mean overcorrection with the higher treatments of +3.36 diopters (SD 0.75) in the 3 diopter group and +4.40 (SD 1.05) in the 4 diopter

Table 8–2. Refraction Over Time (All Patients)

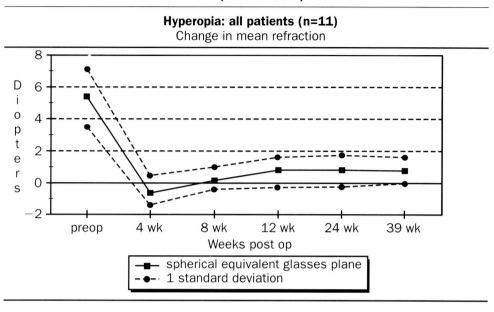

Table 8–3. Refraction Over Time (2D Attempted Correction)

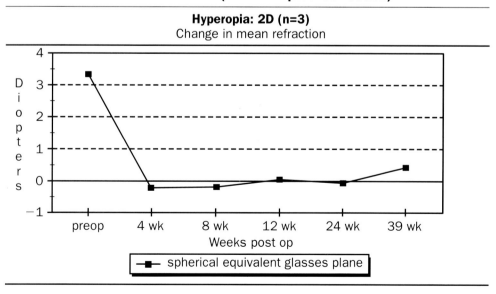

Table 8–4. Refraction Over Time (3D Attempted Correction)

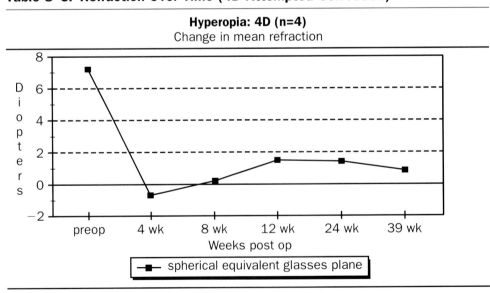

Table 8–5. Refraction Over Time (4D Attempted Correction)

group. In both the 3 and 4 diopter groups, there followed a period of regression before refraction appeared to stabilize between twelve and twenty-four weeks.

Mean keratometry data steepened from a preop 42.12 diopters (SD 1.59 D) to a mean of 47.04 diopters (SD 2.70) at four weeks before stabilizing at a mean of 45.17 diopters at twenty-four weeks (SD 3.05). Keratometry as measured by computer-assisted video topography showed a similar initial overcorrection with a mean preop of 42.72 (SD 1.43), steepening to 46.50 at four weeks (SD 2.10) before tending to stabilize at twenty-four weeks with a mean value of 44.70 (SD 2.72). Table 8–6 shows the change in mean manual keratometry for the overall group and Tables 8–7 to 8–9 show the change in mean manual keratometry for the individual groups treated with 2.0, 3.0 and 4.0 diopters of correction. Table 8–10 shows the change in mean computer-assisted video topography for the overall group and Tables 8–11 to 8–13 reveal the changes in mean topography for the individual 2.0, 3.0 and 4.0 diopter treatment groups. Even though these are small numbers of individual patients, it can be seen that the overall figures correlated with refraction showing an initial overcorrection with subsequent regression. The regression tended to continue for

twenty-four weeks in contrast to twelve weeks by refraction. Breakdown of the keratometry data for individual groups shows that although the regression trend in the 3 and 4 diopter treatment group followed the overall trend, the 2 diopter group tended to stabilize earlier, at about twelve weeks. The keratometry figures consistently showed a smaller overall change than the refraction figures. The initial overcorrection measured by manual keratometry and topography was less than that measured by refraction, and furthermore, by twenty-four weeks, the keratometry mean data approximated more closely than refraction the attempted treatment end point.

Induced astigmatism was calculated by vector analysis utilizing an IBM compatible computer and software (ASSORT). Both magnitude and axis of induced astigmatism were assessed taking into account existing astigmatism. This was calculated from keratometry and refractive data. There was +0.75 diopters of approximately 'with the rule' cylinder induced, by refraction, and approximately 1.0 diopter of 'with the rule' astigmatism induced on keratometry data.

Best corrected spectacle visual acuity was 6/6 in the 10 phakic patients and 6/9 in the aphakic patient prior to treatment. No patient dropped

Table 8–6. Keratometry Over Time (All Patients)

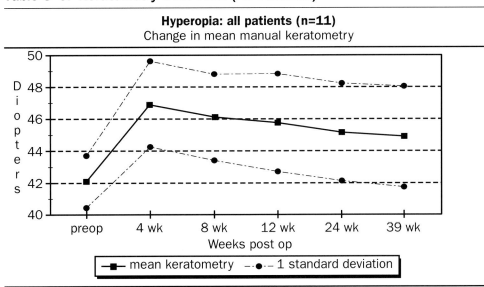

Table 8–7. Keratometry Over Time (2D Attempted Correction)

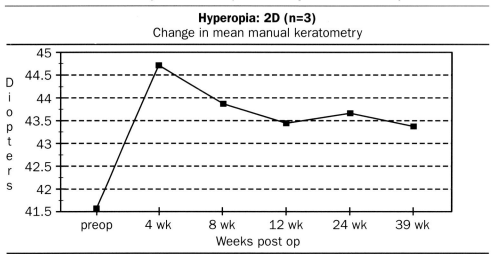

more than two lines on the Snellen chart at any time, although there was certainly a drop in best corrected acuity at the one-month level due to transient induced irregular astigmatism. By nine months all patients had returned to their best corrected visual acuity and one patient had gained one line.

Corneal haze was noted in all patients in an annular ring between 6.5 mm and 8.0 mm, as expected at the site of deepest ablation. This was not felt to be visually significant in any patients and had faded to a trace in all patients by nine months. Haze was more evident in the higher treatment groups.

CONCLUSIONS AND FUTURE PLANS

Our Summit experience using the combination hyperopic mask and Axicon lens to create a mid peripheral trough with a total ablation zone of 9.4 mm appears extremely promising, but also raises significant questions.

This early data suggests that the procedure is safe, but there are some patients who lose best corrected visual acuity for a period of one to two months due to irregular astigmatism. In the patients in this trial and all our subsequent patients, this has

Table 8–8. Keratometry Over Time (3D Attempted Correction)

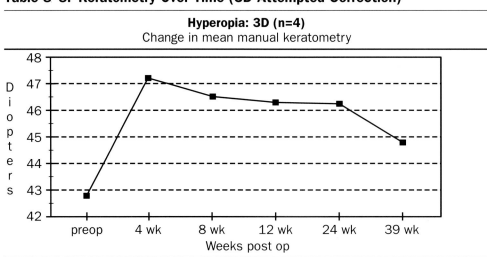

Table 8–9. Keratometry Over Time (4D Attempted Correction)

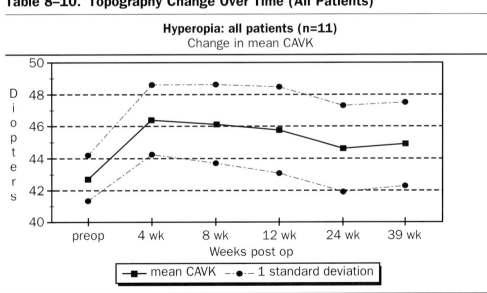

never persisted, but it is possible that there may be a very small incidence of permanent induced irregular astigmatism once a larger cohort have been operated.

Clearly the accuracy of the procedure needs to be refined. At the moment the labeled correction of 2.0, 3.0 and 4.0 diopters are producing an overcorrection. The degree and extent of this overcorrection needs to be further analyzed and the algorithms and number of programmed Axicon pulses refined.

Regression of refractive effect is present at all ranges and stabilizes more quickly with the lower corrections. This is a disadvantage though, and delays operating on the second eye. It would be a significant advance if the initial overcorrection was able to be modified to enable a faster end point to be achieved. The refractive stabilization at around three months, and the keratometric and topographic stabilization at around six months has not been explained, but it suggests that true stability is

Table 8–10. Topography Change Over Time (All Patients)

Table 8–11. Topography Over Time (2D Attempted Correction)

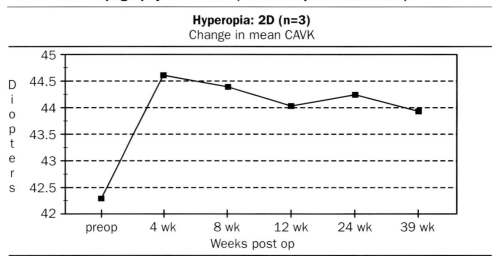

still not certain. The tables indicate that the procedure seems stable after six months, but it will probably take 18 months to two years to be certain of stability in this procedure. This should be viewed cautiously as the main limiting factor for hyperopic PRK corrections in the past has been the regression of intended effect which continues beyond six and twelve months.[3] It may be that the Summit technique has solved this problem, and it certainly appears so, but this has not been conclusively proven from our data at this stage.

It is interesting to note that keratometry and topography measurements are closer to the chosen treatment parameters than the spherical equivalent refraction. The reason for this is unclear, as is the discrepancy between refraction and keratometry, whereby the induced change in hyperopia is greater on refraction than keratometry (which is the same as that seen in myopes). We have previously detailed that in myopic PRK correction, particularly in high myopes, the induced change on spherical equivalent refraction is greater than that seen on

Table 8–12. Topography Over Time (3D Attempted Correction)

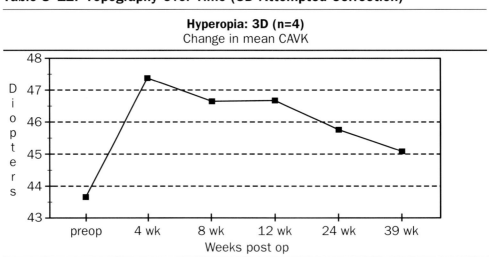

Table 8–13. Topography Over Time (4D Attempted Correction)

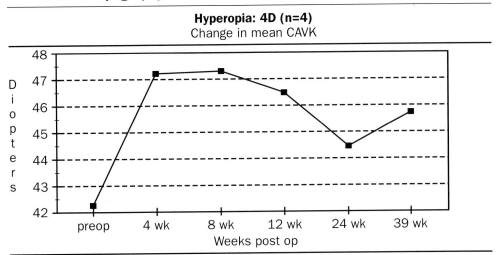

keratometry.[4] We have previously postulated a number of mechanisms, and why this trend should be observed in hyperopic corrections is unclear.

The induced astigmatism as measured by vector analysis showed a slight 'with the rule' induction and this vertical steepening was an unexpected finding. This was apparent both on keratometry and refraction. It is possibly due to lid pressure whereby the removed trough of tissue in the mid periphery causes some corneal ectasia and lid pressure then causes a vertical steepening. This does seem to be a permanent change and will need to be closely followed.

The mid peripheral haze observed was not of concern to either observers or patients and faded with time as seen in myopic PRK. As it is away from the visual axis it is reassuring, but at the same time it raises a question. Since the ablation at its widest point occurs reasonably close to the limbus, is there any potential damage to the limbal stem cells? If this occurs, it would be of considerable concern regarding ocular surface health. This would be a difficult assessment to measure and may not become apparent for many years.

One of the difficulties in assessing hyperopic treatment is what parameters to measure. The usual parameters of corrected and uncorrected visual acuity and what is happening on the cornea in terms of keratometry, topography and corneal clarity are obtained in the normal manner. The difficulty is that, unlike myopic corrections, unaided visual acuities are less useful as an indicator of patient satisfaction and/or surgical success. This is because of the age range of the treated patients and their variable residual accommodation. It is interesting that, of the patients we have treated both in this series and in increased numbers over the last six months, patient satisfaction with this procedure seems extremely high. This may be related to the fact that a hyperopic patient beyond the age of 35 to 40 years has no point in space at which they are appropriately in focus without correction (unlike myopic patients who at least have some point in space where they are in focus without correction). Any reduction in a hyperope's refractive error is an improvement, whereas the myopic patients have a focal point to refer to in terms of comparing their unaided visual acuity. This is a chance observation and it would be difficult, using patient's satisfaction criteria, to establish whether there is a difference in perception between hyperopic and myopic patients in this regard.

As LASIK becomes a more commonly used procedure around the world for myopia and myopic astigmatism, it will be difficult to apply these large ablation zone techniques beneath a LASIK flap. It may be that beneath a LASIK flap, a large ablation zone is not an essential requirement. Although at this stage, the concept of a large ablation zone with a greater blend zone in the mid periphery appears to offer the best chance of refractive success with hyperopic corrections and medium-term stability.

How this could be transposed to the concept of LASIK is unclear at this stage.

In conclusion, with the Summit combination mask in rail and Axicon lens system we have a treatment option for hyperopia which appears safe, capable of correcting up to approximately six diopters, and is relatively stable after three to six months. A larger controlled cohort of treated patients will allow refinement of the algorithms and help explain the as yet unanswered questions surrounding the procedure.

REFERENCES

1. Lawless MA, Rogers C, Cohen P: Excimer laser photorefractive keratectomy: 12 months follow up. *Med J Aust* 159:535–538, 1993.

2. Seiler T, Wollensak J, et al: Myopic photorefractive keratectomy with the excimer laser. One year follow up. *Ophthalmology* 98:1156–1163, 1991.

3. Daush D, Kelin RJ, Schroder E, et al: Excimer laser photorefractive keratectomy for hyperopia. *Refract Corneal Surg* 9:20–28, 1993.

4. Rogers CM, Lawless MA, Cohen PR, et al: Photorefractive keratectomy for myopia of more than −10 diopters. *J Refract Corneal Surg* 10 (suppl)S171–173, 1994.

CHAPTER 9

Photorefractive Keratectomy for Hyperopia:

VISX Experience

Colman R. Kraff
W. Bruce Jackson
Marc G. Odrich

INTRODUCTION

Since the late 1980s, VISX Inc. (Santa Clara, CA) has manufactured excimer laser systems for the treatment of myopia and myopic astigmatism. In the United States, VISX received approval from the Food and Drug Administration (FDA) in January 1996 for the treatment of low to moderate myopia. Clinical trials for myopic astigmatism have been completed. Treating myopia and astigmatism, however, only covers approximately one half of the population with refractive errors. The population of patients with hyperopic refractive errors is estimated to be as large a potential pool of patients (if not larger) than those with myopic refractive errors.[1] Treating hyperopia with an excimer laser, however, raises an entirely different set of problems for the laser manufacturer and refractive surgeon to overcome.

In order to correct hyperopic refractive errors, the central cornea needs to be steepened. Excimer laser technology uses the process of photoablation—removal of tissue. Treating hyperopia therefore becomes a tremendous challenge. How can we steepen the cornea by removing tissue? The answer lies in changing the shape of the peripheral corneal surface while leaving the central cornea untouched. In this chapter, we will review the method by which VISX is currently utilizing the *Star Excimer Laser System* for the correction of hyperopia or H-PRK.

THE VISX STAR EXCIMER LASER

When designing a new excimer laser system for the treatment of hyperopia, VISX attempted to utilize their existing technology, while at the same time incorporating new technology for corneal steepening. The *Star* laser utilizes VISX's dual diaphragm system for the treatment of myopia and myopic astigmatism. A hyperopia module is added along the laser pathway for corneal steepening procedures. Although hyperopic PRK is still investigational in the United States, all *Star* lasers are designed so the hyperopia module can be easily added to any system.

Before beginning a discussion of the hyperopia module specifically, a brief discussion of the basic functions of the *Star Excimer Laser System* in general is appropriate.

The *Star* system is designed to remove corneal tissue in a clean precise manner using the process of ablative photodecompensation. As in other excimer laser systems, the VISX *Star* system uses the rare gases argon and fluorine that when combined and excited, produce an ultraviolet wavelength of 193 nm. The *Star* laser delivers this energy with precision using a computer-controlled delivery. The raw energy in the laser cavity is greater than 400 mJ/cm^2. By the time the beam reaches the corneal plane, the energy is approximately 160 mJ/cm^2. The laser's firing rate is set at 5 Hz with capability of up to 30 Hz[2].

The laser is controlled by the VISX *VisionKey* software. This software utilizes an optical memory card. This card is a WORM (write once read many) device that allows the system operator to program the specific refractive corrections for each individual patient. All myopic and myopic astigmatic treatments with the *VisionKey* software are limited to a maximum 6.0 mm optical zone diameter. The system is capable however of treating up to a 6.5 mm optical zone of treatment for myopic ablations.[2]

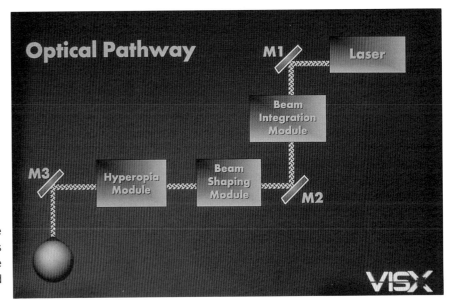

Fig. 9–1. Schematic diagram of the laser pathway. Note the three mirrors and the relationship between the mirrors, the rotating hex prisms and the hyperopic module.

The *Star* system design has reduced the number of mirrors from six (as in the original VISX Twenty Twenty model B) to three mirrors. The laser incorporates two rotating hex prisms between mirror #1 and mirror #3 in order to temporally integrate, and thereby smooth, the shape of the beam to improve quality. The hyperopia module is placed between mirror #2 and mirror #3 (Fig. 9–1). Additionally, the *Star* system incorporates new software that allows the system to automatically calibrate itself by checking fluence and alerting the system operator when potential problems may arise. This increased automation, improved beam quality, and increased mirror efficiency has allowed VISX to add technology to the system with the capability of producing steeper corneas (as opposed to only flatten corneas).[3] Ultimately this will have benefits for patient and surgeon alike.

Hyperopic Ablation

The hyperopic module is added to the laser path between mirrors #2 and #3 (Fig. 9.1). The module directs the excimer beam through a rotating wheel with a series of annular apertures of decreasing width (Fig. 9–2). As mentioned previously, the cornea needs to be steepened in order to correct hyperopic refractive errors. This is achieved by ablating more tissue from the mid-peripheral cornea than the central cornea.

In order to achieve this affect, ablation profiling is provided by rotating an eccentric lens, combined with a rotating variable-width slit mechanism, both of which are under computer guidance. The width of the slit, the offset of the eccentric lens, and the angle of rotation of both the lens and the slit jaws are synchronously controlled through computer software (Fig. 9–3). The module is calibrated to correct an optical zone of 5.0 mm with a transition zone out to 9.0 mm diameter. The deepest area of ablation is at the 5.0 mm diameter and is approximately 10 microns tissue per diopter of correction. The depth of ablation decreases centripetally and centrifugally from the 5.0 mm diameter. The central 3.0 mm of the optical zone remains untouched (Fig. 9–4).

The desired refractive change, the ablation depth per pulse, and the average keratometry readings for the patients are entered into the *VisionKey* software (in a similar manner to that of myopic patients. For each patient, a test block of plastic is ablated to ensure calibration. The resulting plastic refractive change is verified by a lensometer. If the resultant lensometer reading is different than the desired refractive correction, the energy calibration of the laser is adjusted using the appropriate calibration

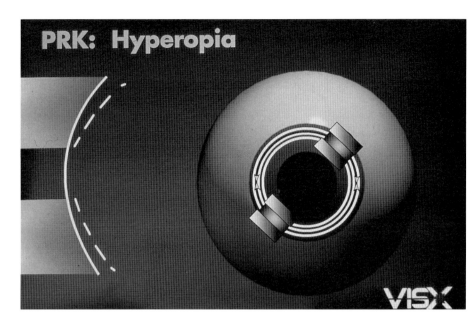

Fig. 9–2. Schematic of the cornea with the rotating wheel apertures.

factors that are provided with the VISX software. Once the desired lensometer reading is achieved, patient treatment can be initiated.

CURRENT SURGICAL TECHNIQUE

The patient may be given systemic medication (analgesic, sedative) at the physician's discretion prior to the procedure. A topical anesthetic is placed in the operative eye. A lid speculum is placed into position. The fellow eye is patched to insure good fixation with the operative eye. The operative eye is aligned so the projected reticule is centered on the center of the entrance pupil (Fig. 9–5), while the patient fixates on a blinking red fixation light. The zone over which the ablation is going to occur is marked using a 9.0 mm optical zone marker. The epithelium is then removed mechanically to a diameter of 11.0 mm. The surgeon then refocuses on the anterior corneal surface. The reticule is then recentered over the patient's pupil and the patient is asked to reaffirm that they can see the red fixation light. The foot pedal is depressed and the surgery is performed. During the procedure, the surgeon is able to actively track the patient and insure centration by using the *Star* joystick control system throughout the procedure.

Immediately following the procedure, the eye is patched and the patient is given the appropriate pain medication. The patient is seen daily until the corneal surface has reepithelialized.

CLINICAL RESULTS (U.S. AND CANADA)

Partially Blind Eye Trials

To the best of our knowledge, at the time of writing this chapter, VISX is the only company that has initiated H-PRK clinical trials in North America. The first human clinical trials for hyperopia were initiated in the U.S. by VISX in the summer of 1993. This was a Phase I FDA clinical trial of ten partially signed blind eyes. The VISX Excimer Laser System model B was modified so the excimer beam was directed through a wheel with a series of annular apertures of decreasing width similar to that described above. The mean age of the ten patients was 55.4 years +/− 18.8 years with a range of 29.7 to 91.0 years at the time of treatment. Six patients were male and four were female. No patients best corrected spectacle visual acuity was better than 20/100 preoperatively. Nine of the ten patients were examined at 12 months. One patient was lost to follow-up after eight-month postoperative visit. A

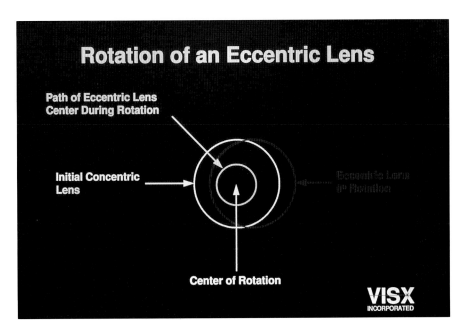

A

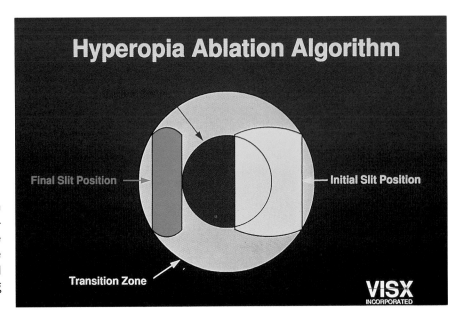

B

Fig. 9–3. Drawing of the ablation algorithm profiles showing the pattern that is produced using the eccentric lens. 3A: Schematic of the eccentric lens positions. 3B: Initial and final positions of the rotating blades.

second patient suffered a filamentary keratitis that in the opinion of the operating surgeon, was unrelated to the surgery as it had been present for several years prior to the treatment. There were no other serious adverse events or complications.

The patients were all screened for serious corneal pathology. All patients were examined by the refrac-

tion, corneal topography, slit lamp examination, dilated fundus examination and intraocular pressure monitoring at the preoperative, one-month, three-month, six-month and twelve-month visits postoperatively.

A 4.0 diopter correction was attempted in all patients. Because the patients visual acuity ranged

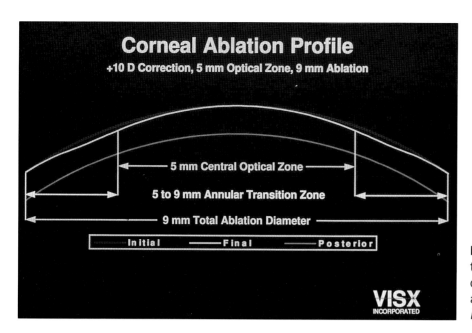

Fig. 9–4. Schematic representation of the corneal shape and optical zone sizes after a hyperopic ablation with the *Star Excimer Laser System*.

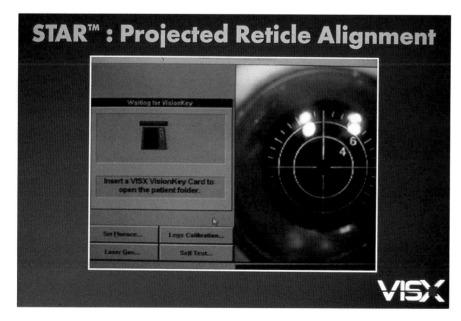

Fig. 9–5. Heads up display with the virtual projected centering reticule. This is the actual view that the surgeon sees through the operating microscope.

between 20/200 to hand motion, the reliability of postoperative data measurements is limited. Half of the patients were treated with a 8.0 mm optical zone and half with a 9.0 mm optical zone.

Results of Preliminary Trials

Results of nine of the ten patients at one year demonstrated adequate safety and efficacy to warrant a phase II trial. No patient had a significant loss of preoperative best corrected spectacle visual acuity (BCSVA), although the patients were partially sighted preoperatively. There was no significant corneal haze. Patients treated with the 9.0 mm ablation algorithm appeared to be more stable over time than those treated with the 8.0 mm ablation algorithm. Videokeratography demonstrated central corneal steepening which appeared stable.

These results were within an acceptable level of safety and efficacy to justify further clinical trials in sighted eyes. These Phase II trials were started in the summer of 1995 at the University of Ottawa Eye Institute, Ottawa General Hospital. Our co-author, Dr. W. Bruce Jackson, is the principal investigator for this ongoing trial.

Patient Selection Criteria

The inclusion criteria for the trial were as follows: Patients had to be 21 years of age or older with stable hyperopia for one year between +1 to +4 diopters spherical equivalent with less than 1D of cylinder. The best corrected visual acuity had to be 20/40 or greater in each eye. Contact lens wear had to be stopped two to four weeks prior to final evaluation with stable keratometry. Patients with any serious medical condition, on any systemic medication affecting healing, with any active ocular

Table 9–1. Spherical Equivalent Results of PRK-H

		Hyperopia PRK Results		
Visit	Num	Mean SE	SD	Mean Haze
Preop	25	+2.48	±0.90	0
1M	25	−0.35	±0.52	0.26
2M	25	−0.10	±0.62	0.38
3M	24	+0.09	±0.54	0.31
4M	4	+0.44	±0.38	0.50

disorder, or with a history of prior eye surgery were excluded from the study. Women who were pregnant or lactating were also excluded from the study.[4] The surgical technique was similar to that described above.

Surgical Results

A total of 25 patients (25 eyes) were treated, of which 15 were female and 10 were male. The mean age was 50 years (Range 39-62). The mean spherical equivalent was +2.48 diopters with a mean astigmatism of +0.59 diopters. The epithelium was healed in 13 patients at day #3 and 11 patients at day #4. One patient was healed at day #6. The change in mean spherical equivalent (SE) over time can be seen in Table 9–1. At the 3-month visit the SE was 0.09 D +/− 0.54 D. A comparison of the preoperative versus the postoperative uncorrected visual acuity (UCVA) can be seen in Table 9–2. Preoperatively, 36% of the patients had an UCVA or 20/40 or better. At the 3-month postoperative visit, 92% of the patient had an UCVA of 20/40 or better. Refractive results demonstrated that at the

Table 9–2. Uncorrected Visual Acuity Results

		Star Hyperopia UCVA				
Visit	Num	20/10 20/20	20/25 20/40	20/50 20/100	20/25 or better	20/40 or better
Preop	25	4%	32%	64%	16%	36%
1 Month	25	28%	60%	12%	64%	88%
2 Month	25	40%	52%	8%	60%	92%
3 Month	24	50%	41%	8%	71%	92%
4 Month	4	25%	75%	—	25%	100%

Table 9–3. Refractive Results

Hyperopia Results

Visit	Num	±0.5 D	±1.0 D	−1.1 to −2.0 D	+1.1 to +2.0 D
1 Month	25	68%	92%	8%	—
2 Month	25	76%	88%	8%	4%
3 Month	24	75%	96%	—	4%
4 Month	4	50%	100%	—	—

3-month visit, 96% of the patients were with $+/-$ 1.0 D of emmetropia (Table 9–3). Loss of best corrected visual acuity (BCVA) was also evaluated in this group of patients. At the 3-month visit, 54% of the patients had zero lines lost of BCVA, while 46% had loss of one line of BCVA (Table 9–4). No patients lost two or more lines of BCVA by the 3-month postoperative visit.[5]

Complications

Complications were evaluated in two categories: those related to complications from healing, and those complications related to visual symptoms. Table 9–5 lists those complications related to postoperative healing. The majority of the complications are related to epithelial healing problems. The most common complications were epithelial erosions documented in 12 of 25 patients. Haze was graded as 0.5 or less in 21 of 25 patients. Visual complications are listed in Table 9–6. One hundred percent of the patients were very well pleased or pleased with the results.[5]

Table 9–4. Percent Loss of BCVA

Hyperopia Line Loss of BCVA

Visits	Num	0	1	2	3
1 Month	25	48%	40%	12%	—
2 Month	25	64%	32%	4%	—
3 Month	24	54%	46%	—	—
4 Month	4	25%	75%	—	—

Table 9–5. Medical Complications

Hyperopia Complications

• Delayed Wound Healing (6 Days)	1/25
• Corneal Surface Irregularities	
Filaments	5/25
Epithelial erosions	12/25
Epithelial ridge	5/25
• Peripheral Marginal Infiltrate	1/25
• Haze 0.5 or less	21/25
• Arcuate scar	1/25

Table 9–6. Visual Complaints

Hyperopia Complications

• Visual Symptoms	
Tailing	3/25
Shadowing/haloes/double-vision	3/25
Blurred vision	2/25
Letters packed together	1/25
Photophobia	3/25

Table 9–7. Subjective Evaluation

Hyperopia Subjective Evaluation

Very pleased with results	68%
Pleased with results	32%
Unhappy with results	0%

DISCUSSION

Since the early 1990s, excimer laser surface PRK for myopia in the low to moderate range has become the surgical procedure of choice as an alternative to contact lenses and glasses in the international arena. In the United States—with the approval in 1996 PRK for low to moderate myopia—the trend will probably mirror that of our international colleagues.

Treating hyperopia with the excimer laser raises an entirely new set of questions that need to be answered with respect to safety and efficacy. Some of these questions are similar to those that we encountered early on in myopic PRK. Optical zone size, ablation depth, regression and haze all appear to play a role in producing accurate safe results in hyperopic excimer correction. VISX has attempted to address some of these questions with the ongoing clinical trials to date.

After completion of the partially blind eye phase I FDA trial, modifications were made to the ablation algorithms, treatment zone size, surgical technique, and hardware. These modifications are reflected in the results from the Canadian trials at the University of Ottawa. The 3-month postoperative results in general are very good. The procedure appears to have good safety in the small cohort of normally sighted eyes. The efficacy is still being evaluated. The ablation algorithms have demonstrated fairly good accuracy, yielding good UCVA and reduction of hyperopic refractive error. There were no vision threatening complications and no patient lost two lines or more of their previous best corrected visual acuity. As this ablation produces a minification of the image, it is anticipated that a small percentage of loss of BCVA may occur, but this should not be on the order of two lines of visual acuity. These, however, only reflect limited data on a small cohort of patients over a short period of time. These patients will need to be followed care-

fully over the next several months to determine if regression, haze formation, or late postoperative complications occur.

Additionally, VISX plans to start a multicenter U.S. trial on a larger cohort of patients. Similar inclusion and exclusion criteria will be used in the U.S. clinical trial. Ultimately, the results of these clinical trials will yield data that will tell us if PRK-H is a viable alternative for glasses and contact lenses in this patient population, as PRK is in the myopic population.

REFERENCES

1. Projected Population Vision Correction Devices by Age and Spherical Distribution, 1986–1992. Health Products Research, 1989.
2. VISX Operators Manual, 1996. VISX Inc., Santa Clara, CA.
3. Terrance Clapham, Ph.D., Senior Vice President Research and Development, VISX, Inc. Santa Clara, CA. (Personal Communication).
4. VISX Clinical Protocol for PRK-H at the University of Ottawa Department of Ophthalmology. Ottawa, Canada.
5. Jackson WB, Mintsioulis G, Agapitos PJ, et al: Excimer Laser Surgery for the Correction of Low to Moderate Hyperopia with the VISX Star Excimer Laser System. Pacific Coast Refractive Symposium. Whistler, B.C., Canada, February 15–19, 1996.

CHAPTER 10

Photorefractive Keratectomy for Hyperopia

Experience with the Nidek EC 5000

Hugo Sutton
Sally Donaldson

INTRODUCTION

The benefits of the Nidek EC 5000 scanning laser for surface ablation as established in myopic and astigmatic treatments include improved epithelial healing times, less regression, and a lower instance of haze compared with outcomes from the VISX 20/20B. The Nidek EC 5000 laser can be utilized for H-PRK.

METHODS

Hyperopic and associated myopic cylindrical photoablations were performed on 29 eyes using the Nidek EC 5000 scanning laser, pictured in Fig. 10–1. The software version was 2.20 initially, then 2.23. The mean preoperative spherical refraction was +4.43 diopters (range +0.75 to +8.5), and the mean cylindrical refraction was 2.30 diopters (range 0 to −5.50). The treatment zone for the myopic astigmatic correction was 6.5 mm with a blend zone to 7.5 mm, and for the hyperopic correction was 5.0 mm to 5.5 mm with a transition zone out to 9.0 mm. For the initial software, overcorrection was planned using an in-house algorithm of sphere and minus cylinder, adding between 10% and 20% of the minus cylindrical power that was fully treated on top of the hyperopic component. For the 2.23 version of the software, the full sphere plus the minus cylinder was used. Standard post-operative PRK drop regimen was used including FML starting qid after re-epithelialization, and tapering 1 drop every 4 weeks.

RESULTS

Re-epithelialization

Re-epithelialization time was 3 to 5 days. Three patients took up to 9 days to re-epithelialize from their primary treatment.

Uncorrected Visual Acuity

At three months 90% had uncorrected vision of 20/40 or better, and 100% had best corrected vision of 20/25 or better. *See* Fig. 10–2.

Best Corrected Spectacle Visual Acuity

At three months postoperative 64% had no loss of best corrected visual acuity and 36% had a one line loss of best corrected vision. No patients showed loss of two or more lines of best corrected acuity. See Fig. 10–3.

Change in Refraction

The changes in refraction after surgery are outlined in Fig. 10–4. Two weeks post-operative the mean spherical component was +1.30 diopters (range −1.0 to +4.5) and the cylindrical component was −0.67 diopters (range −0.25 to −2.5). One month postoperative, the mean spherical component was +1.75 diopters (range −2.0 to +5.5) and the cylindrical component was −0.86 diopters (range 0 to −2.0). Three months after surgery the mean spherical component was +2.55 (range −0.5 to +4.75) and the cylindrical component was −0.93 diopters (range 0 to −1.75).

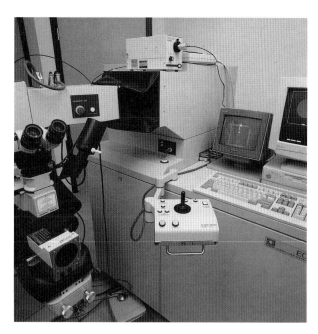

Fig. 10–1. Nidek EC 5000 excimer laser.

Topographic Changes

The central cornea is steepened as shown in Fig. 10–5. Fig. 10–6 shows a postoperative central steep area in an elevation type map using the ORBSCAN machine. Preop, three week and four week maps are shown.

Corneal Haze

At one month postoperative 75% had trace or no haze, 15% had grade 1 haze, 10% had grade 2 haze and no patients had grade 3 haze. At three months postoperative 90% had trace or no haze, and 10% had grade 1 haze.

DISCUSSION AND CONCLUSIONS

All hyperopic treatments are compelling from a patient's perspective. Following treatment some patients experienced an unpredicted ability to see well at both distance and near in spite of being well into the presbyopic age group. This may be due to the positive asphericity of their resultant cornea.

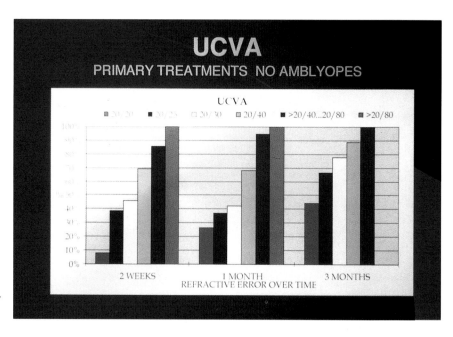

Fig. 10–2. Uncorrected visual acuity over time; 90% 20/40 or better.

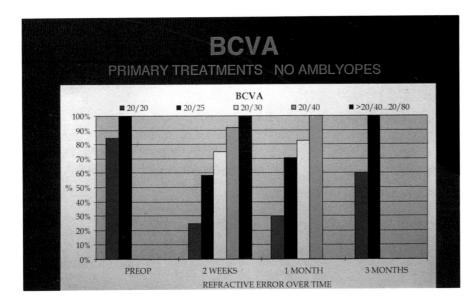

Fig. 10–3. Best corrected visual acuity over time; 100% 20/25 or better at 3 months.

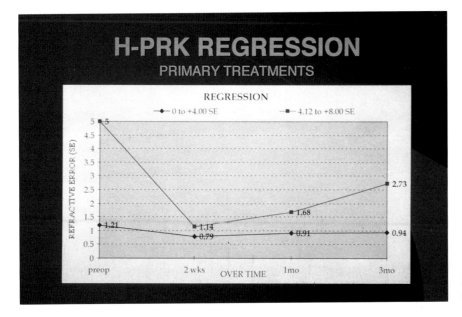

Fig. 10–4. Refractive error regression over time.

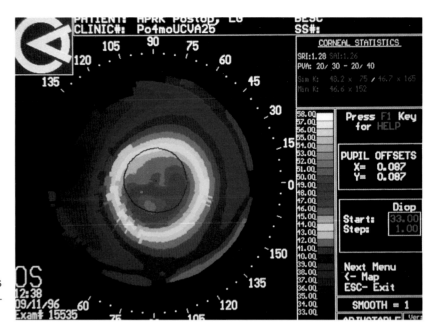

Fig. 10–5. Curvature map 4 months post H-PRK; note steepening of the central cornea.

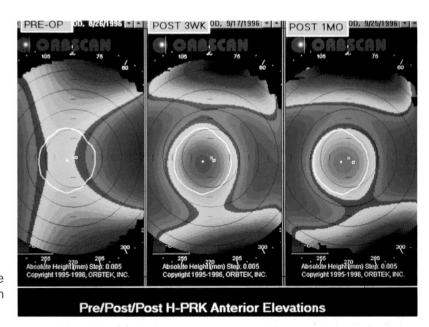

Fig. 10–6. Anterior elevation difference map; note increased anterior elevation centrally.

The prolonged re-epithelialization rate may lead to increased haze. The reasons for delayed re-epithelialization include not just the wide ablation zone, but the resultant steepness of the central cornea. As with other hyperopic surface systems, those treatments with less than 4 diopters seem to have much better predictability and stability than treatments of greater than 4 diopters. Nonetheless, the few treatments carried out above 7 diopters of hyperopia that provided a lasting effective treatment are evidence of the potential of this technology. The problems of delayed re-epithelialization and high chance of enhancement in the higher powers in particular lend credence to the idea of carrying out LASIK as a primary treatment.

section III

Photoablation for Hyperopia and Presbyopia

B. Non-excimer Laser

CHAPTER 11

The Correction of Hyperopia Using the Novatec Solid State Laser

Casimir A. Swinger
Shui T. Lai

INTRODUCTION

Surface photorefractive keratectomy (PRK) for the correction of low to moderate myopia has been shown to be safe and efficacious.[1] In addition, toric surface PRK and LASIK (laser in situ keratomileusis) for correction of myopia and astigmatism also appear very promising. The past and current major challenges of refractive surgery are the correction of hyperopia and presbyopia.[2–16] Although lamellar refractive surgery, in the form of hyperopic keratomileusis, has long been used to successfully correct hyperopia, the technique is cumbersome and accompanied by technical difficulty.[3,13,16] With the exception of a few investigators the use of the excimer laser for the correction of hyperopia has had limited application and success, primarily because of the difficulty in achieving a satisfactory ablation profile with large diameter.[2,10] The Novatec solid state laser has been developed to address the limitations of excimer laser technology and, in this chapter, we will describe its use for the correction of hyperopia.[14,15]

THEORY

To correct hyperopia, the central cornea must be steepened. As seen in Fig. 11–1, this necessitates a corneal trough, or aspheric blend zone, in the midperiphery to reduce the regression that would accompany a vertical wall at the outside boundary of the ablation. This may be achieved by direct reprofiling of the anterior corneal surface (surface PRK) or by stromal ablation following a lamellar keratectomy (LASIK). Even though such a contour is physically achievable, it may produce unacceptable clinical results if the total diameter is too small or the blend zone not appropriately designed. Also,

if the pupil dilates beyond the optic zone proper, there is the possibility of visual symptoms if the optic zone is not wide enough, the ablation not well centered, the pupil large, or any combination thereof.

INSTRUMENTATION

Microkeratome

The lamellar keratectomy in LASIK is performed with an electromechanical microkeratome.[17] Although any microkeratome, such as the classic Barraquer and BKS (Barraquer-Krumeich-Swinger) devices may be used, a motorized unit is usually used to provide a more uniform passage across the eye. Although the costs of the motorized devices are significantly greater, there have been, unfortunately, no controlled comparative studies comparing accuracy and surface quality. Most units allow the surgeon to vary the depth of the keratectomy via some mechanical means, although in LASIK the keratectomy is typically standardized at approximately 130–160 microns, depending on the correction. Microkeratomes that allow only a fixed depth should allow for greater safety and less risk of inadvertent penetration into the eye. For hyperopic LASIK it would appear ultimately desirable to have a resection diameter as large as 10–11 mm to accommodate a large ablation diameter without ablating the hinged flap.

Novatec Solid State Laser

Reprofiling of the cornea is accomplished with ultraviolet (UV) photoablation. Although most UV lasers can reprofile the cornea to effect central steepening, they vary considerably with respect to how this is accomplished and also with respect to

Novatec Hyperopia Protocol

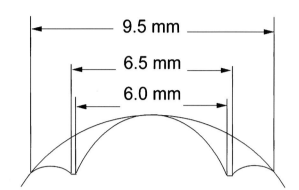

Fig. 11–1. Hyperopic surface PRK profile following ablation.

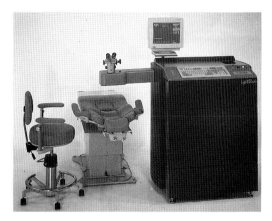

Fig. 11–2. Novatec solid state "LightBlade" laser.

the profiles and ablation diameters that are physically achievable, which can be the final arbiters of success or failure.

Lasers differ in their delivery systems. Early lasers used circular or slit-shaped broad beam 6–7 mm) delivery systems that distributed laser energy with the assistance of apertures, diaphragms, or masks. A requisite for success in hyperopic PRK (H-PRK) is an ablation diameter significantly larger than that typically used for myopic PRK to allow for the peripheral aspheric blend zone that will join the maximum depth of ablation at the edge of the optic zone proper to the corneal surface in the periphery. Laser manufacturers have accomplished this in different ways, such as with a linear broad scanning slit and an eye mask having a spiral-dash shaped aperture,[2] wide area ablation in conjunction with a special mechanical modification to increase the ablation zone diameter[10] and two-step ablation, where the optic zone is ablated first to an optic zone of 6.5 mm followed by a second step whereby the laser energy is optically redistributed and only the periphery ablated to produce the aspheric blend.

The authors have previously presented a new technology for photorefractive keratectomy using a computer directed "flying spot" scanning delivery system, the Novatec "LightBlade" laser (Fig. 11–2).[14] The laser uses no gases but only solid state laser crystals to achieve a wavelength in the deep ultraviolet part of the spectrum. The laser parame-

ters, when used for the correction of hyperopia, are as follows: wavelength: 0.21 microns; fluence: 100 mJ cm[2], delivery system: computer-directed "flying spot" scanning; spot size: adjustable from 0.10–0.50 mm (typically used at 0.20–0.30 mm); optical zone: unlimited (spherical optic zone of 6.5 mm and total ablation diameter of 9.5 mm typically used for hyperopic PRK; toric ablations use a 6.0 mm × 6.0 mm optic zone with an additional 1.25 mm taper at each end of the scanned axis for a final dimension of 6.0 mm × 8.5 mm).

The Novatec laser operates in a single fundamental mode with a gaussian spatial energy distribution and has excellent pulse-to-pulse stability. The nature of the surgical beam precludes the possibility of hot or cold spots, thus requiring no homogenization optics and lessens the number of optical components subjected to UV damage. Because the surgical beam is collimated, there is no strict requirement that the microscope be exactly focused on the surface to be ablated. That is, the fluence at the cornea is independent of microscope adjustment. Also, the patient and surgeon lines of sight are coaxial with the patient fixation beam and the surgical laser beam itself, allowing for a perfectly centered ablation.

The Novatec laser employs a computerized "flying spot" scanning delivery system that we believe is important to allow truly customized ablation profiles, whether to produce specific peripheral aspheric blend zones, or to correct concomitant asymmetric or even irregular astigmatism. Currently, the scanning pattern is concentric-circular for spherical corrections and linear for toric corrections, but it may be programmed to any pattern. Any complex algorithm may be programmed to allow for surface reprofiling. In the near future, topographic data from the cornea will be inputted into the system and energy delivered by computer control to achieve the desired ablation profile. One may liken the laser to a computer-directed "light pen", whereby any profile may be generated after computer entry at the keyboard. In addition, a remote maintenance module using a modem can be used for data entry.

Because of the small spot size and low fluence, the Novatec laser places much less energy on the cornea at any given instant when compared to typical excimer lasers. For example, using the Novatec laser with a 0.2 mm spot size and a 100 mJ/cm^2 fluence reduces by hundreds of times the energy at any moment when compared to a broad beam excimer laser with a 6 mm optic zone and a fluence of 150 mJ/cm^2, thus resulting in no audible sound during the ablation, less acoustic shock waves and reduced trauma to the eye.

The Novatec laser system uses an active eye tracker, which functions equally well in surface PRK or LASIK, that redirects the surgical beam should any eye movement within a range ±5 mm (10 mm diameter) take place. The eye racker is extremely rapid, and the beam position is updated every two milliseconds. We believe that an eye tracker is important for H-PRK, because the procedure time is typically prolonged compared to a comparable myopic correction. More importantly, the eye tracker should assist in reducing decentration of the optic zone, should there be any eye displacement during ablation. This is much more important in H-PRK or hyperopic LASIK than for myopic PRK, as a small decentration will bring the aspheric mid-peripheral area within the pupillary zone and may result in secondary image formation that may be bothersome to the patient or even reduce visual acuity.

PRECLINICAL STUDIES

The authors and coworkers performed hyperopic surface ablation with the Novatec laser on both enucleated bank eyes and in a nonhuman primate model following ablation profile studies in enucleated porcine eyes. Based on these studies, it appeared that an optic zone of 6.0–6.5 mm with a total ablation diameter of 9.0–9.5 mm appeared to produce a satisfactory topographic pattern. Following the development of an algorithm, H-PRK was performed on four nonhuman primate eyes. A correction of 5.00 D was requested in each instance. The results indicated that a stable hyperopic correction was achievable.

CLINICAL STUDIES

Based on the preclinical studies, a limited human trial of H-PRK and hyperopic LASIK was initiated in Canada and Mexico (R) with Donald Johnson, M.D., Howard Gimbel, M.D., Erik Williams, M.D., and Arturo Chayet, M.D., and the early results have been recently presented.[15] The study is limited to low to moderate hyperopia with a range of spherical equivalent of 0.50 D to 7.00 D and a refractive cylinder of 0.75 to 5.00 D, which may be treated along with the hyperopia. Patients must be a minimum of 21 years of age, are allowed to have had previous corneal surgery, and the treated eye must be free of other ocular pathology, although they are allowed to have mild amblyopia. See Table 11-1.

The current protocol calls for a central optic zone of 6.5 mm, which may be single or multizone depending on the optic correction desired, beyond which is a mid-peripheral blend zone with an outer ablation diameter of 9.5 mm (Fig. 11–1). The first several eyes in the series were treated with a 9.0 mm diameter ablation, but this was soon increased to 9.5 mm. Congenital hyperopes tend to have corneas of smaller diameter than normal, and a peripheral cuff of epithelium should be left intact to expedite epithelialization of the corneal surface. Thus, although the ablation zone can be made as large as desired by the laser, there is a practical limitation in the hyperopic eye. Of course, a consecutive hyperope who was previously myopic before other surgery can accommodate a larger ablation diameter.

To date, 24 eyes that have been entered into the H-PRK study are at least one month postoperative. The maximum follow-up at this time in any eye is one year, although many eyes have only recently undergone surgery. Although we have been evaluating myopic LASIK for some time, we have only recently begun study of hyperopic LASIK and the follow-up is currently too short to report at this time.

SURGICAL TECHNIQUE

Hyperopic Surface PRK

The surgical procedure is similar to myopic surface PRK and begins with topical anesthesia followed by manual removal of the corneal epithelium. The corneal diameter had first been measured, and the debridement is carried out to the far periphery, to approximately 10 mm, while maintaining a small residual cuff of epithelium at the limbus. The patient then fixates on the coaxial fixation beam of the Novatec laser and centration is further assured by the reticle in the eye piece and the two guiding beams that are focused on the cornea and seen near the pupillary margin. Laser ablation is then carried out after first engaging the eye tracker to maintain centration.

Following surgery, patients are treated with a nonsteroidal drop, an antibiotic and a bandage lens. Patients are seen regularly until epithelialization is complete.

Postoperatively, patients are prescribed a topical antibiotic, nonsteroidal, and fluorometholone (FML) 0.1% drops until epithelialization is complete, at which time the bandage lens is removed and the patient thereafter treated with topical FML t.i.d. for one month. The topical steroid is tapered according to a schedule, depending on the refractive result at the one month evaluation.

Hyperopic LASIK

For hyperopic LASIK, the keratectomy is performed with any commercially available microkeratome, using a resection depth of 160 microns and the largest available diameter. Until now we have used the Automatic Corneal Shaper (Chiron Ophthalmics, Inc., Irvine, CA) that has provided a resection diameter of approximately 8.5 mm. In such cases we alter the ablation profile to an optic zone of 5.5 mm and an ablation diameter of 8.5 mm. We are currently evaluating newer microkeratome models in order to achieve a larger resection diameter. The management of the LASIK patient is similar to that of the H-PRK patient, except that the bandage lens is removed in 24 hours and all medications are stopped after the third postoperative day.

RESULTS

As is seen, patients included six overcorrected myopic surface PRK's and four failed Ho:YAG laser thermal keratoplasties (LTK's). In addition, this series includes what we believe to have been the first reported case of an overcorrected radial keratotomy patient. At the time of surgery the LTK patients, though they had undergone significant regression, had achieved reasonable stability following their regression postoperatively and still had a residual correction.

Epithelialization following H-PRK is expected to be more lengthy than following myopic surface PRK. A 10 mm zone of debridement results in a 78.5 mm^2 defect as compared to a 6 mm zone, which is only 28.3 mm^2. Nevertheless, the mean epithelialization time was 4.52 days. Patients were sometimes not seen between the third and seventh

Table 11–1. Refractive History

Number	History
13	Congenital hyperopia
6	Overcorrected myopic PRK
4	Regressed Ho:YAG laser thermal keratoplasty
1	Overcorrected radial keratotomy
—	
24	

Table 11.2. Refractive Change Following Hyperactive PRK

	3 Months	6 Months
N	16	8
Pre	+3.34 D	+5.22 D
Post	+0.41 D	+1.47 D
Change	−2.93 D	−3.75 D

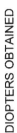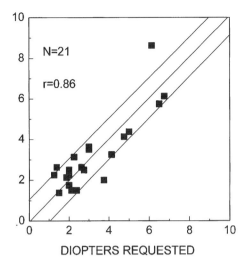

Fig. 11–3. Scattergram of hyperopic PRK at one month.

days, and this figure thus represents a conservative value. For seven eyes followed daily, the mean closure time was 3.4 days. These values are quite satisfactory considering the large epithelial defect and the fact that contact lenses and nonsteroidal anti-inflammatory agents (NSAID's) were used, which are believed to delay epithelialization.

For 16 eyes at three months, the mean hyperopic spherical equivalent of +3.34 D was reduced to +0.41 D, whereas for eight eyes at six months the mean hyperopia of +5.22 D was reduced to +1.47 D (Table 11–2). With respect to accuracy in achieving the desired refractive correction (Figs. 11–3, 11–4), 38% of eyes at one month were within ±0.50 D, and 86% of eyes were within ±1.00 D of intended correction, though this latter figure was 63% at three months, and will be discussed under stability. Small overcorrections would leave the person slightly nearsighted and presumably happy as opposed to an overcorrected myopic patient who became hyperopic. Thus, the algorithm may be adjusted to give a slight overcorrection.

There was a small but statistically significant decay of the achieved correction between the first and third months postoperatively, with the mean refraction at one month of +0.02 D decreasing to +0.50 D for 15 eyes (Fig. 11–6). This may reflect some epithelial hyperplasia in the aspheric blend zone or simply be the result of stabilization of the optic zone with its epithelial cover. One eye was significantly overcorrected (2.50 D) at one month and contributed most to the mean observed regression. This eye has remained near emmetropia from the second to sixth months, however. For five eyes between the third and sixth months, the refraction was perfectly stable with a mean change of +0.01 D during this interval. However, for three eyes that

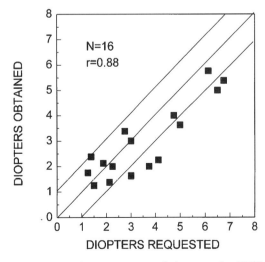

Fig. 11–4. Scattergram of hyperopic PRK at three months.

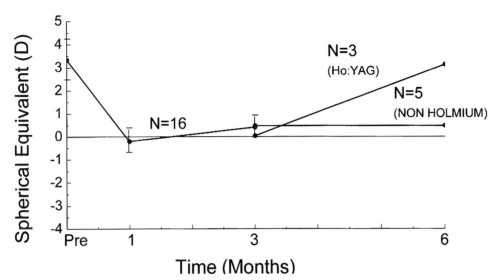

Fig. 11–5. Stability following hyperopic surface PRK with the Novatec Laser.

had had previous Ho:YAG laser thermal keratoplasty, there was a significant regression (2.05 D) between the third and sixth months, for which there may be several reasons. First, the previous surgery may have altered the corneal collagen in a way that leads to greater instability following H-PRK, which removed Bowman's membrane in the region. The H-PRK procedure also removes an area of tissue most affected by the LTK procedure. Second, the eyes had not fully regressed following LTK, and some of the regression may represent continued LTK regression as opposed to post-H-PRK regression. Lastly, these three eyes had the largest attempted corrections (mean 5.88 D) and were the only eyes treated with a 9.00 mm ablation diameter, rather than 9.5 mm as we now perform the surgery. The small sample size and large number of variables do not allow for definitive conclusions at this time, though further evaluation is indicated in post-LTK treated eyes. In the remainder of the eyes, the relatively good accuracy and stability in the early postoperative phase is very encouraging, although patients must be followed for a longer period of time to demonstrate that the final corrections obtained are stable before the algorithm is modified.

There was no significant increase in the refractive cylinder. The mean preoperative cylinder of 0.63 D was increased by 0.04 D at three months in eyes not treated for cylinder. There is always the possibility of induced astigmatism with H-PRK, as the total ablation time can be lengthy in high corrections, and any decentration of the ablation zone could lead to induced astigmatism. The use of the eye tracker in these cases allowed for good centration and no induced astigmatism.

Visual recovery following H-PRK appears somewhat slower than following myopic PRK. Preoperatively, 76% of eyes had a best-corrected acuity of 20/25 or better and 90% had 20/40 or better. At one month postoperatively (Table 11–3), 24% had 20/25 or better uncorrected acuity and 67% had 20/40 or better. These figures increased to 44% 20/25 or better and 75% 20/40 or better at three months. At three months, when best-corrected acuity is still improving, 38% of eyes gained one or more lines of best-corrected visual acuity, 1996 lost one line, and 5% lost two lines (Table 11–4). It must be remembered that unlike surgery for myopia, which results in a larger retinal image postoperatively and is often accompanied by an improvement in best-corrected acuity for this reason, surgery for hyperopia reduces the image magnification afforded by spectacles, resulting in a smaller retinal image. Historically, surgery for hyperopia has typically been accompanied by minor reductions in

Table 11.3. Uncorrected Acuity Following Hyperopic PRK

	BCVA	1 Mo	3 Mos
	(Pre-Op)		
Number of Eyes	24	21	16
20/25 or Better	76%	24%	44%
20/40 or Better	90%	67%	75%

Table 11.4. Change in Best Corrected Acuity Following Hyperopic PRK

	No Change	Gain 1+ Lines	Lost 1 Line	Lost 2 Lines
1 Month	43%	19%	14%	24%
3 Months	38%	38%	19%	5%

best-corrected acuity for this and other reasons.[3,13,16]

Corneal haze following the procedures was minimal. Haze was observed in 52% of eyes at any time, peaked at three months, and was seen only in the periphery, thus having no visual significance. The mean haze was 0.21 at one month, 0.33 at three months and 0.19 at six months. The maximum haze in any eye at any time was 1.0.

Corneal topography showed that the ablations were well centered, and there was no evidence of central islands or other abnormalities at any exam. Figure 11.5 shows the pre, post and change in

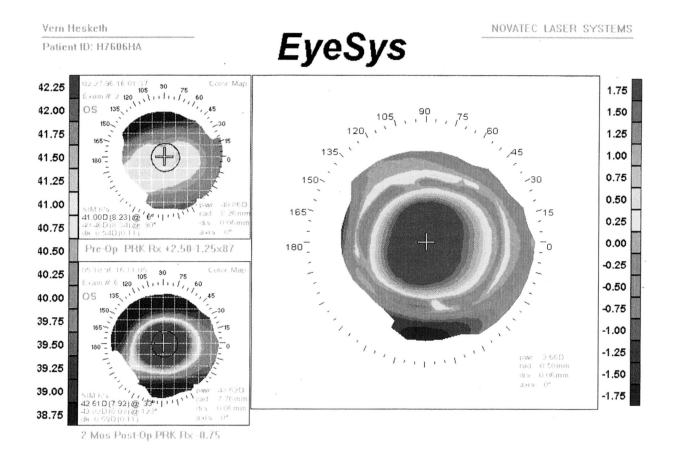

© 1995 EyeSys Technologies Version 3.1

Fig. 11–6. Corneal topography following hyperopic surface PRK with the Novatec laser.

corneal topography following an ablation for a thermal keratoplasty correction.

There were no intraoperative or postoperative complications in this series.

DISCUSSION

Early studies of excimer laser ablation for correction of hyperopia demonstrated the possibility of significant subjective symptoms and regression when smaller optic zone diameters were used,[2] and this has also been seen in the past by following hyperopic keratomileusis (CAS, unpublished observations). Such symptoms have never been noted after having performed hundreds of cases of keratophakia for hyperopia, however. In keratophakia, a tissue addition technique, the corneal curvature does not have the degree of concavity or abnormal mid-peripheral contour as in keratomileusis, H-PRK or LASIK for correction of hyperopia. It is evidence that for the latter procedures the optic zone proper should probably be at least 6 mm in diameter, if not greater. In the future, aspheric optical zones or a multizonal approach may allow the surgeon to increase the size of the optic zone while limiting the ablation depth, and hence profile induced distortion, and procedure time. Only further clinical investigation will allow the determination of the best profile in each case to achieve the most satisfactory results with a minimum of subjective side effects.

In this first study using a new technology with a computerized scanning delivery system and active eye tracker, the Novatec laser, the initial results appear very promising. The accuracy of the correction obtained compared to that requested is very good in the early postoperative period, indicating that the algorithm employed is accurate. It is important to note that in this series a 10 mm debrided zone will epithelialize in a timely fashion. This is important for possibly reducing haze and minimizing infection or other complications. It should be noted also that many eyes in this series had had previous surgery. The ablation characteristics in eyes that have previously undergone photorefractive keratectomy or other refractive surgery may not be equivalent to primary cases. In addition, some patients had laser thermal keratoplasty or radial keratotomy, and the refractive results and the sta-

bilities obtained must be evaluated in the light of these previously performed procedures, which may still have been generating a biomechanical action. Nevertheless, the results demonstrate the safety and initial efficacy of photorefractive keratectomy using surface ablation for the correction of hyperopia, congenital or consecutive.

Certainly, if the intended correction is low, disturbance in the corneal profile and contours is minimized, and one would expect the results to perhaps be more efficiently attained than high hyperopic corrections. Nevertheless, corrections up to 6.00 D were obtained in this series without significant side effects. Only further clinical investigation will demonstrate the long term safety and effectiveness of this approach when compared to performing the hyperopic ablation on the stromal bed following an initial lamellar keratectomy in the form of a LASIK procedure. The latter, of course, will still provide similar challenges with respect to corneal contour changes at the anterior corneal surface, along with increased cost, technical complexity, demand for greater skill on the part of the surgeon and the typical complications seen in lamellar surgery, such as epithelial ingrowth.

In conclusion, laser refractive surgery for the correction of hyperopia, long a challenge, is now on the threshold of success. This will finally offer to the hyperopic patient, whether a congenital hyperope or, worse, a consecutive hyperope following previous unsuccessful surgery, the benefits experienced by the myopic population.

REFERENCES

1. Salz JJ, Maguen E, Nesburn AB, et al: A two-year experience with excimer laser photorefractive keratectomy for myopia. *Ophthalmology* 100:873–882, 1993.
2. Anschütz T: Laser correction of hyperopia and presbyopia. *Intl Ophthalmol Clin* 34(4):105–135, 1994.
3. Barraquer JI: Keratomileusis for myopia and aphakia. *Ophthalmology* 88:701, 1981.
4. Dausch D, Klein R, Landesz M, et al: Photorefractive keratectomy to correct astigmatism with myopia or hyperopia. *J Cataract Refract Surg* 20(suppl):252, 1994.
5. Dausch J, Klein R, Schröder E: Excimer laser photorefractive keratectomy for hyperopia. *Refract Corneal Surg* 9:20–28, 1993.

6. Dausch D, Landesz M: The Aesculap-Meditec excimer laser: results from Germany. In: Salz JJ, McDonnell PJ, McDonald MB (eds): *Corneal Laser Surgery*, St. Louis, CV Mosby, 1995, p 237–247.

7. Ditzen K: LASIK experience in myopia and hyperopia including cylindrical corrections. Abstracts of the ASCRS symposium on cataract, IOL and refractive surgery, April 1–5, 1995, p 27.

8. Jensen R: Hexagonal keratotomy; clinical experience with 483 eyes. *Int Ophthalmol Clin* 31:69–73, 1991.

9. Kaye GB, Gimbel HV, van Westenbrugge JA, Deschenes MC: Early outcomes of photorefractive keratectomy for hyperopia using 3 different laser systems. *Inv Ophthalmol Vis Sci* 37(3):S55(abstract), 1996.

10. Macy JI, Nesburn AB, Salz JJ: VISX blind eye study United States results. In: Salz JJ, McDonnell PJ, McDonald MB (eds): *Corneal Laser Surgery*, St. Louis, CV Mosby, 1995, p 256–260.

11. Méndez-Noble A, Méndez A: Flap and Zap for the treatment of primary hyperopia. Abstracts of the ASCRS symposium on cataract, IOL and refractive surgery, April 1–5, 1995, p 21.

12. Ramirez-Florez S, Koons SJ, Shimmick JK, et al: Correction of hyperopia with excimer laser PRK. *Invest Ophthalmol Vis Sci* 35(4):2023(abstract), 1994.

13. Swinger CA, Barraquer JI: Keratophakia and keratomileusis—clinical results. *Ophthalmology* 88:709, 1981.

14. Swinger CA, Lai ST: Solid state photoablative decomposition—the Novatec laser. In Salz JJ, McDonnell PJ, McDonald MB (eds): *Corneal Laser Surgery*, St. Louis, CV Mosby, 1995, p 261–267.

15. Swinger C, Lai S, Johnson D, Gimbel H, Lai M, Zheng W: Surface photorefractive keratectomy for correction of hyperopia using the Novatec laser. *Inv Ophthalmol Vis Sci* 37(3):S55(abstract), 1996.

16. Troutman RC, Swinger CA: Refractive keratoplasty-keratophakia and keratomileusis. *Trans Am Ophthalmol Soc 76:329, 1978.*

17. Pallikaris IG, Papatzanaki ME, Siganos DS et al: A corneal flap technique for laser in situ keratomileusis. Human studies. *Arch Ophthalmol* 109:1699–1702, 1991.

section IV
Lamellar Techniques

CHAPTER 12

Automated Lamellar Keratotomy (ALK) for Hyperopia

David R. Hardten

INTRODUCTION

The desire to gain increased independence from the use of glasses and contact lenses is not unique to the myope. Certainly, the hyperope and presbyope share these desires. These patients have increasing dependence on their glasses and contact lenses as they age because of the loss of accommodation. For many of these patients, refractive surgery is a reasonable alternative. Lamellar refractive keratotomy for hyperopia was developed from the concepts and work of Dr. Jose Barraquer in Bogota, Columbia.[1,2] The procedure is termed a keratotomy because the tissue is incised, but no tissue is removed.[3] Hyperopic cryolathe keratomileusis and epikeratoplasty can reduce hyperopia, but are associated with significant loss of best-corrected spectacle acuity.[4–7]

Luis Ruiz, M.D., has also been a pioneer in this area and noted that a deep lamellar pass can reduce hyperopia. This has been refined through development of the microkeratome until this procedure can now be used to correct hyperopia with relative accuracy. This procedure, though, is relatively new and the long-term effects are still not known. More study needs to be performed before the relative indications for hyperopic automated lamellar keratotomy are known as compared to other surgical corrections for hyperopia such as hexagonal keratotomy, epikeratoplasty, photorefractive keratectomy, phakic intraocular lenses, lens extraction with intraocular lens implant, radial thermokeratoplasty, or holmium laser keratoplasty.[4–29]

HISTORICAL REVIEW OF CURRENT TECHNIQUE

Drs. Jose Barraquer and Luis Ruiz have had great influence on the development and advancement of keratomileusis.[1,2,29–31] Dr. Ruiz discovered while performing keratomileusis that, if the procedure was aborted before the cryolathe was used to reshape the corneal lenticule, the eye actually became more myopic. This led to development of nomograms for the correction of hyperopia.[20,21,22,30–33]

The effects of freezing on the cornea have been associated with a prolonged healing process that may result in corneal edema and therefore many different systems have been developed to try to add or remove tissue from the eye without necessitating freezing the tissue.[34–43]

The results of keratomileusis *in situ* for myopia are significantly dependent on the accuracy of the microkeratome used. The depth, as well as the smoothness of the cut, are extremely important. In most of the early systems, the speed of the keratome moving across the eye was dependent on the surgeon. A very fast movement creates a thinner cut than a very slow movement.[44]

Because of this variability, in the late 1980s Luis Ruiz developed an automated geared keratome that controlled the speed of the pass across the eye so that more consistent lamellar resections were possible. Improvements in the suction ring have increased the ease of the procedure and the keratectomies with this newer device are smoother than with previous instrumentation. These facts have led to increasing use of the microkeratome.[45]

PRINCIPLES OF HYPEROPIC AUTOMATED LAMELLAR KERATOTOMY

Automated lamellar keratotomy for hyperopia causes ectasia of the central cornea creating steepening that can reduce hyperopia. The goal in this ectatic procedure is to reproducibly produce a defined amount of ectasia that remains stable following the procedure. Hexagonal keratotomy is another

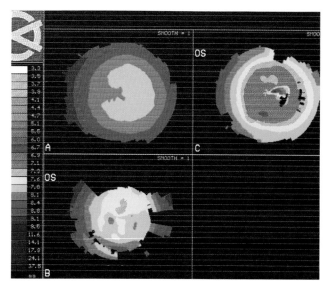

Fig. 12–1. Computerized corneal topography following automated lamellar keratotomy for hyperopia. The central cornea is steeper than before the procedure. (A) Preoperative topography, (B) Two weeks after hyperopic ALK, and (C) Three weeks after hyperopic ALK.

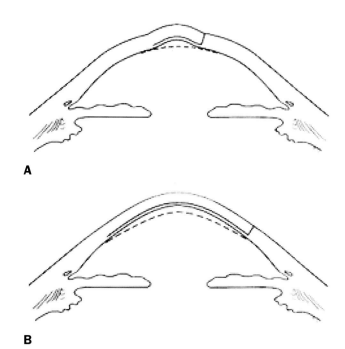

Fig. 12–2. The central corneal bows anteriorly as the deep lamellar cut causes ectasia. If this occurs over a relatively small area, the central corneal curvature is greater (12–2A) than when the ectasia occurs over a larger area (12–2B).

procedure that reduces hyperopia through central corneal ectasia, but unfortunately is not reproducible or stable.[9–10,15] Topographic changes of the cornea from hyperopic automated lamellar keratotomy result in an aspheric surface that is steeper in the center and flatter in the periphery (Fig. 12–1).

This steepening is quite obvious immediately after the initial microkeratome cut removes a thick section of cornea. With the cap removed, a thin layer of posterior stroma remains in position. The intraocular pressure then causes this thin flap of remaining tissue to protrude forward. The anterior cap maintains this steeper curvature when it is placed back over the deep lamellar cut, reducing or eliminating hyperopia.

The amount of ectasia that occurs is dependent upon the optical zone of the area of ectasia. When ectasia occurs, the cornea becomes forwardly displaced. If this occurs over a small area, the curvature is relatively high (Fig. 12–2A). When this ectasia is spread out over a larger optical zone, then the amount of steepening that occurs at any one spot is less (Fig. 12–2B).

It is important to have a deep enough lamellar cut to produce ectasia, but the surgical effect is dependent less on the depth of the cut than it is on the optical zone diameter. To gain ectasia, a cut of 60–80% depth is necessary. There is an increased probability of progressive ectasia with deeper cuts, and so the current recommended depth of cut is 60–65% of the central corneal thickness.

Luis Ruiz, M.D., developed the initial nomogram for correction of hyperopia with the automated corneal shaper, and this has been modified by Lindstrom, Casebeer, Hollis and Rozakis to allow for higher corrections (Table 12–1).

CRITERIA FOR PATIENT SELECTION

Over 120 million Americans are currently dependent on glasses or contact lenses and therefore may be potential candidates for refractive surgical procedures—with even more potential candidates worldwide.[46] Appropriate indications for hyperopic

Table 12–1. Nomogram for Correction of Hyperopia with Automated Lamellar Keratotomy

Diopters (Spherical Equivalent)	Optical Zone (mm)
1.0	6.6
1.5	6.5
2.0	6.4
2.5	6.3
3.0	6.2
3.5	6.1
4.0	6.0
4.5	5.8
5.0	5.6
5.5	5.4
6.0	5.2
6.5	5.0

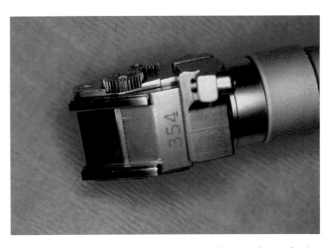

Fig. 12–3. The Automated Corneal Shaper from Steinway/Chiron. The gears allow movement of the shaper head across the cornea at a constant speed.

ALK include hyperopia of a low to moderate degree, a desire to decrease dependence on glasses and contact lenses, appropriate expected outcome, good ocular health, and a normal cornea. Patients who have had previous radial keratotomy or hexagonal keratotomy are not good candidates because they are at a much higher risk of progressive corneal ectasia from excess weakening of the cornea.

PATIENT OBJECTIVES AND PREOPERATIVE MANAGEMENT

In patients in the presbyopic age group, an appropriate discussion of whether the patient desires distance or near vision is important. Manifest and cycloplegic refractions are helpful to uncover any latent hyperopia. Computerized topographical analysis of the corneal surface should be performed to rule out sub-clinical keratoconus or other corneal diseases. Appropriate educational materials should be given to the patient, and an extensive informed consent discussion should occur between the patient and surgeon.

INSTRUMENTATION

Many different microkeratomes have been used in the past for lamellar resection of the cornea.[30,45,47–58] Currently, the most commonly used

microkeratome for correction of hyperopia is the Automated Corneal Shaper by Steinway (Miami, Florida) and Chiron (Claremont, California), (Fig. 12–3). This microkeratome is unique in that it has gears that pull it across the cornea at a constant speed. All microkeratomes work on the same principle as a carpenter's plane. Tissue is fed between a protective block and the moving blade, allowing cuts of a relatively precise thickness.[59]

The suction ring has an adjustable portion to allow variability in the diameter of corneal tissue to be resected (Fig. 12–4). The applanation lens is scored to allow precise control of the diameter of tissue resected. A stop on the microkeratome head can be adjusted to allow the blade to stop before the cap is entirely removed[60] (Fig. 12–5). All parts must be meticulously cleaned and cared for to allow proper movement of the parts.

SURGICAL PROCEDURE

Topical anesthesia is used. Typically, three drops of proparacaine are used. Too much anesthetic can lead to loosening of the epithelium that can then be retained in the interface. Occasionally, sedation such as diazepam may be necessary. The patient is centered underneath the operating microscope after appropriate preparation with Betadine is performed. A lid speculum is used to separate the eyelids. The visual axis is marked with a 5 mm optical

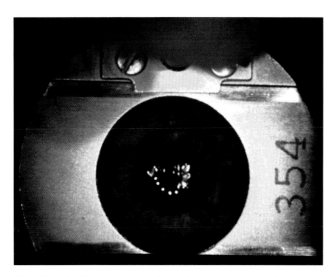

Fig. 12–4. The suction ring of the automated corneal shaper is adjustable to allow various resection diameters. As the rings collapse closer together, the diameter of the cut enlarges.

zone marker. An additional mark is made temporal to the visual axis to assist in alignment of the flap. Central corneal pachymetry is measured. Sixty to 65% of the central corneal thickness is then calculated to determine the intended depth of resection. The appropriate block is then placed in the microkeratome head. It is important to have the stop set to the hyperopic setting.

The suction ring of the automated corneal shaper is then brought into place. The suction rings are opened to the approximate amount needed for a resection of the appropriate optical zone before being placed on the eye. The suction ring is centered on the pupil and the optical zone mark (Fig. 12–4). Careful centration is crucial because of the relatively small optical zone used.

The suction is then turned on. A tonometer is used to make certain that the intraocular pressure has been raised to above 65 mm Hg. The applanation ring is used to make certain that the diameter of the flap is set to the intended resection size. Smaller optical zones will result in larger degrees of correction.

During the measurement of the resection diameter, it is crucial that the corneal epithelium be dry to allow accurate measurements. The adjustment wrench is then removed from the suction rings. The automated corneal shaper (with a plate attached to create the appropriate depth cut) is then brought into place. The microkeratome is passed across the cornea in an automated fashion (Fig. 12–6). A small hinge is used to prevent dislocation of the flap. The

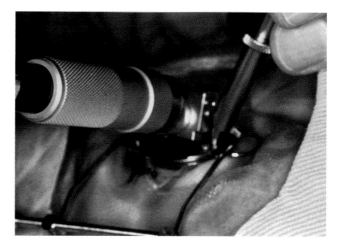

Fig. 12–6. The keratotome is positioned in the track and is mechanically moved across the cornea by the gears, cutting a lamella of tissue with thickness limited by the distance between the metal block and blade. It is important to make certain the proper thickness block is positioned securely in the keratotome. If the block is loose or left out, a cut much deeper than intended can occur.

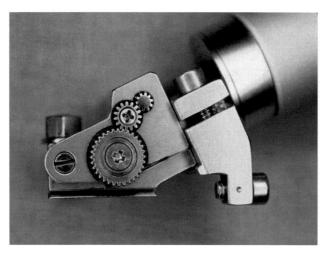

Fig. 12–5. The stop is set even with its holder for myopia, but for the shorter hyperopic cuts must be partially extended.

corneal shaper and suction ring are removed from the eye. Any remaining debris is removed from the stromal surface. A single drop of BSS is placed on the stromal bed and the flap is floated into position. The flap is smoothed over with a wet Merocel sponge and any debris is carefully removed from the eye.

The flap is allowed to dry into position for five minutes with the lid speculum still in place, providing time for the endothelial cell pump to remove stromal fluid from underneath the flap, securing it into position. The lid speculum is removed and the patient is allowed to blink, assuring that the flap remains in position. The patient's eye may be taped closed if it is felt that there is any chance the flap may move. Antibiotic, steroid, and nonsteroidal drops are again instilled at the end of the case. No contact lens is used as these patients are quite comfortable even on the first postoperative day. A clear plastic bubble protector is taped over the eye.

POSTOPERATIVE MANAGEMENT

Typically, the patient recovers quite rapidly postoperatively. There may be some initial hyperopia followed by progression toward myopia. Antibiotics and steroids can be used two to four times daily for one to two weeks. The patient is seen the first day postoperatively to make certain the flap is in good position. The final refractive result is evident in one to three months.

RESULTS

Short-term results of hyperopic automated lamellar keratotomy have been presented.[18,20–22] Longer follow-up is now available on the eyes from our center.

In this study, 45 eyes with a spherical equivalent between +1.12 and +7.12 D (mean +2.75 ± 1.03 D) had hyperopic ALK. Of these eyes, 35 had no previous corneal surgery and had a spherical equivalent ranging from +1.12 to +7.12 D (mean +3.47 ± 1.56 D) and astigmatism ranging from 0 to 6 D (mean +1.52 ± 1.84 D). Ten of the eyes had previous corneal surgery including seven eyes with prior RK and three eyes with prior photorefractive keratectomy. These eyes had a spherical equivalent ranging from +1.25 to +4.37 D (mean +2.19 ±

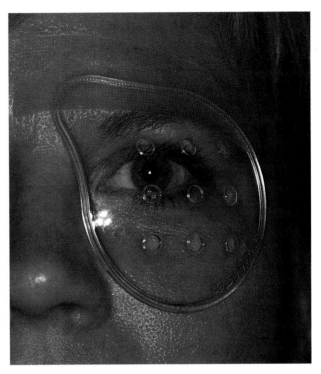

Fig. 12–7. Clear plastic "bubble" eye shield used postoperatively to protect the eye from trauma the first day postoperatively until the flap securely heals into place.

1.02 D) in astigmatism ranging from 0 to 1.50 D (mean 0.96 ± 0.57 D).

The mean pachymetry for all 45 eyes was 550 ± 34 microns. The mean depth of the incision was 367 ± 42 microns (67% of central pachymetry). The mean optical zone size was 6.0 ± 0.4 mm. Ten of the eyes (22%) had simultaneous astigmatic keratotomy for correction of astigmatism.

In the eyes that had no previous corneal surgery, the mean pachymetry was 553 ± 41 microns and the mean depth of cut was 372 ± 41 microns (67% of central pachymetry). The mean optical zone size in these patients was 5.0 ± 0.4 mm. Nine of these eyes (26%) had simultaneous astigmatic keratotomy.

In the patients that had previous corneal surgery, the mean pachymetry value was 540 ± 69 microns. The mean depth of the cut in these patients was 352 ± 40 microns (65% of central pachymetry). The mean optical zone size was 6.4 ± 0.1 mm. One eye (10%) had astigmatic keratotomy at the time of the hyperopic ALK.

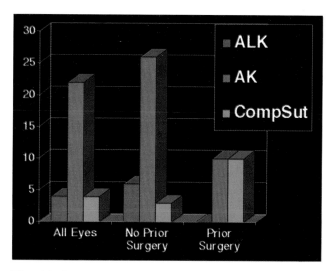

Fig. 12–8. Enhancement rate following hyperopic ALK in all 45 eyes, 35 eyes with no prior corneal surgery, and 10 eyes with prior RK or PRK. Enhancements with ALK are shown in red, enhancements with astigmatic keratotomy in yellow, and compression suture placement in orange.

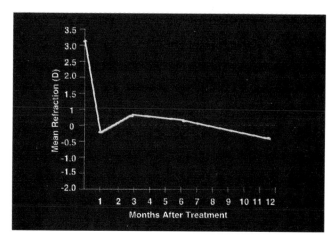

Fig. 12–9. Most of the refractive result in hyperopic automated lamellar keratotomy occurs soon after the surgery. The results are relatively stable in this graph of results in 45 eyes undergoing hyperopic automated lamellar keratotomy. The mean spherical equivalent is plotted versus time.

Enhancement was needed with further ALK in two of the total eyes (4%) and enhancement with astigmatic keratotomy was required in ten eyes (22%), (Fig. 12–8). Compression suture for overcorrection was required in two eyes (4%). The enhancement rate for those patients without previous corneal surgery was 6% for further ALK, 26% for AK, and 3% required a compression suture for overcorrection. In the ten eyes that had previous corneal surgery, one eye (10%) was enhanced with astigmatic keratotomy and one eye (10%) required a compression suture for severe ectasia.

The mean follow-up for all the eyes is 8.6 ± 4.2 months. The mean spherical equivalent at last follow-up is +0.25 ± 1.3 D (range—2.12 to +5.75 D). Most of the correction occurs soon after the procedure (Fig. 12–9). The mean change of best-corrected visual acuity was a loss of 0.12 lines with a range of three lines lost to three lines gained.

In eyes that had previous surgery, the mean spherical equivalent at the last follow-up is −0.25 ± 1.0 D (Range −2.00 to +0.75 D). The mean change is best-corrected visual acuity is +0.14 lines with a range of two lines lost to three lines gained. In eyes

without previous surgery, the mean spherical equivalent at last follow-up is +0.50 ± 1.3 D with a range of −2.12 to +3.12 D. The mean change of best-corrected visual acuity is −0.4 lines with a range of three lines lost to three lines gained.

Of all of the eyes, 28 (62%) are within 1 diopter of emmetropia at the last follow-up (Fig. 12–10). Thirty-five of the eyes (88%) are within 2 diopters of emmetropia. Uncorrected visual acuity is better than 20/40 in 71% of the eyes and better than 20/25 in 29% of the eyes.

In patients that have had previous corneal surgery, six of the eyes (60%) are within 1 diopter of emmetropia and seven eyes (70%) are within 2 diopters of emmetropia at last follow-up (Fig. 12–11). Six of the eyes (60%) had uncorrected visual acuity of 20/40 or better at the last follow-up and two eyes (20%) had uncorrected visual acuity of 20/25 or better at last follow-up. Of eyes without previous corneal surgery, 12 (34%) were within 1 diopter of emmetropia at the last follow-up. Twenty-eight of the eyes (80%) are within 2 diopters of emmetropia at the last follow-up. Twenty-six of the eyes (74%) had uncorrected visual acuity of

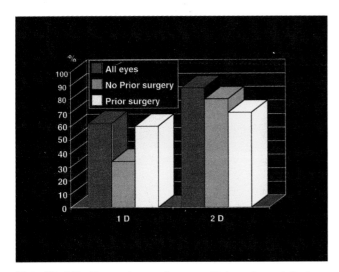

Fig. 12–10. Percentage of eyes within a 1 and 2 diopters of emmetropia after hyperopic automated lamellar keratotomy. All 45 eyes (red bars) are compared with 35 eyes with no prior corneal surgery (yellow bars) and 10 eyes with prior RK or PRK (green bars).

20/40 or better at the last follow-up. Eleven of the eyes (31%) were 20/25 or better at last follow-up without correction.

Epithelium grew into the interface in one eye, but no significant decentrations or cap losses were seen. Irregular astigmatism was very common early after the procedure with decreased best-corrected visual acuity, but improved with longer follow-up.

From the data in this study, it is clear that enhancements are possible in a large number (26%) of patients. The procedure is capable of reducing hyperopia, though, with relative accuracy.

Follow-up of 12 months is available in four of the eyes with previous corneal surgery and in 17 of the eyes without previous corneal surgery. There is a mean drift towards myopia of −0.72 diopters in those patients with previous radial keratotomy or photorefractive keratectomy. This difference between 6 and 12 months is not statistically significant (p = 0.4), but this trend may suggest that these patients are at risk of developing progressive myopia. In the eyes that had not had previous corneal surgery, the difference between the 6 and 12-month spherical equivalent in the 17 patients

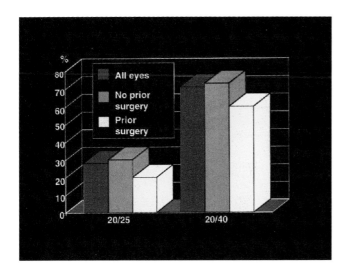

Fig. 12–11. Percentage of eyes with uncorrected visual acuity 20/25 or better and 20/40 or better. All 45 eyes (red bars) are compared with 35 eyes with no prior corneal surgery (yellow bars) and 10 eyes with prior RK or PRK (green bars).

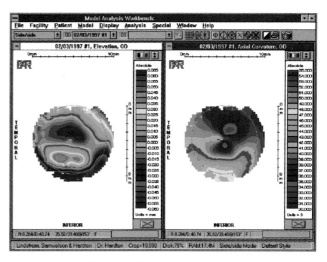

Fig. 12–12. This patient had hyperopic ALK post progressive hyperopia after RK. Severe ectasia is demonstrated by the elevation of the cornea above a best fit sphere present inferiorly (left), with associated steepening and irregular astigmatism (right).

that had follow-up at both the 6 and 12 months was 0 diopters. Therefore this subgroup of patients, with a mean depth of incision of 67% of central pachymetry, did not have any progressive ectasia if they had not had previous corneal surgery.

In another series of hyperopic automated lamellar keratotomy, 24 eyes of 17 patients had ALK using the automated corneal shaper.[22] The mean attempted correction was +3.90 D. Follow-up is available at six months for 17 of these eyes. Seven of the 17 eyes (41%) were within 1 diopter of attempted correction, uncorrected acuity was 20/40 or better in 13 (87%) and 20/20 or better in eight eyes (53%). There was a mean regression towards hyperopia of 0.20 D between one and six months. Two of the eyes (8%) developed clinically significant epithelial ingrowth.

COMPLICATIONS

Complications can occur following any lamellar procedure including hyperopic ALK. A dislocated cap may occur, although this is much less common following hyperopic ALK than after myopic ALK. The thicker flaps are more resistant to dislocation. Proper and careful drying of the flap will decrease the incidence of cap dislocation.[60] If the epithelial integrity is disrupted, the flap may become more edematous and more likely to dislodge. Eye rubbing should be prevented by using a protective shield to prevent mechanical trauma and flap dislocation (Fig. 12–7). The hinge technique has nearly eliminated lost caps.

Melting of the stromal cap can occur over areas of epithelial ingrowth. It is important to remove areas of significant epithelium in the interface to prevent this problem. Retained epithelial cysts or epithelial ingrowth can also lead to significant amounts of irregular astigmatism.

Irregular and regular astigmatism can also occur following hyperopic ALK. Irregular astigmatism tends to improve with time as the flap heals, but if persistent, it may be improved by lifting the flap and repositioning it. Regular astigmatism can be corrected with astigmatic keratotomy.

Under and overcorrection are also possible complications. Residual hyperopia can be treated with repeat ALK for hyperopia or other procedures for hyperopia. Overcorrections with significant levels of

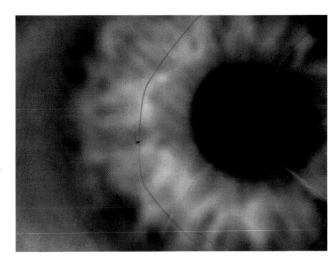

Fig. 12–13. A lasso suture of 11-0 Mersilene can be used to bring radial keratotomy incisions together. This allows reduction in the progressive hyperopia that can occur after radial keratotomy.

undesired myopia can be treated with radial keratotomy, excimer laser photorefractive keratectomy, or placing a running suture in the cap.

Severe ectasia can occur in eyes that have previously undergone procedures that cause ectasia such as radial keratotomy (Fig. 12–12). Compression sutures similar to a lasso are a better option then hyperopic ALK for progressive hyperopia after RK (Fig. 12–13).

Infectious keratitis is extremely rare. Patients must be warned of the early signs of infection and be seen, cultured and treated immediately with antibiotic if this occurs.

All patients have some degree of epitheliopathy because the procedure severs the corneal nerves. Rarely neurotrophic keratitis can occur after hyperopic ALK.

CONCLUSIONS

Hyperopic automated lamellar keratotomy remains a viable alternative to other procedures for the surgical correction of hyperopia. Long-term studies still need to document stability of this procedure. This procedure should not be performed for correction of progressive hyperopia following other procedures that work by causing ectasia such as radial keratectomy.

REFERENCES

1. Barraquer JI: Queratoplastica refractiva est. *Inform Oftal (Inst Barraquer)* 2:10, 1949.
2. Barraquer JI: Queratoplastia. *Arch Soc Am Oftal Optom* 3:147, 1961.
3. Waring GO: Making sense of Keratospeak, IV: Classification of refractive surgery. *Arch Ophthalmol* 110(10):1385–1391, 1992.
4. Arffa RC, Marvelli TL, Morgan KS: Long-term follow-up refractive and keratometric results of pediatric epikeratophakia, *Arch Ophthalmol* 104:668–670, 1986.
5. Barraquer JI: Results of hyperopic keratomileusis. *Int Ophthalmol Clin* 23(3):25–44, 1983.
6. Dingeldein SA, McDonald MB: Epikeratophakia. *Int Ophthalmol Clin* 28:134–144, 1988.
7. McDonald MB, Kaufman HE, Aquavella JV, Purrie DS, Hiles DA, Hunkeler JN, Keates RH Morgan KS, Sanders DR: The nationwide study of epikeratophakia for aphakia in adults. *Am J Ophthalmol* 103:358–365, 1987.
8. Arffa RC, Marvelli TL, Morgan KS: Long-term follow-up of refractive and keratometric results of pediatric epikeratophakia. *Arch Ophthalmol* 106:668–670, 1986.
9. Basuk WL, Zisman M, Waring GO III, Wilson LA, Binder PS, Thompson KP, Grossniklaus HE, Stulting RD: Complications of hexagonal keratotomy. *Am J Ophthalmol* 17:37–49, 1994.
10. Casebeer KC, Phillips SG: Hexagonal keratotomy. A historical review and assessment of 46 cases. *Ophthalmol Clin North Am* 5:727–744, 1992.
11. Charpender DY, Nguyen-Khoa JL, Duplessie M, Colin J, Phillippe D: Radial thermoplasty is inadequate for overcorrection following radial keratotomy. *Refract Corneal Surg* 10:34–35, 1994.
12. Dausch D, Klein R, Landesz M, Schröder E: Photorefractive keratectomy to correct astigmatism with myopia or hyperopia. *J Cataract Refract Surg* 20 (suppl): 252–257, 1994.
13. Dausch D, Klein R, Schröder E: Excimer laser photorefractive keratectomy for hyperopia. *Refract Corneal Surg* 9:20–28, 1993.
14. Durrie DS, Schumer DJ, Cavanaugh TB: Holmium: YAG laser thermokeratoplasty for hyperopia. *J Refract Corneal Surg* 10(suppl):S277–S280, 1994.
15. Ehrlich MI, Nordan LT: Epikeratophakia for the treatment of hyperopia. *J Cataract Refract Surg* 15: 661–666, 1989.
16. Feldman ST, Ellis W, Frucht-Pery J, Anayet A, Brown SI: Regression of effect following radial thermokeratoplasty in humans. *Refract Corneal Surg* 5:288–290, 1989.
17. Foss AJ, Rosen PH, Cooling RJ: Retinal detachment following anterior chamber lens implantation for the correction of ultra-high myopia in phakic eyes. *Br J Ophthalmol* 77:212–213, 1993.
18. Hardten DR, Schneider TL, Parker PJ, Lindstrom RL: Correction of hyperopia using automated lamellar keratoplasty (ALK). *Invest Ophthalmol Vis Sci* 36: S852, 1995.
19. Lyle WA, Jim GJ: Clear lens extraction for the correction of high refractive error. *J Cataract Refract Surg* 20(3):273–276, 1994.
20. Kezirian GM, Gremillion CM: Automated lamellar keratoplasty for the correction of hyperopia. *J Cataract Refract Surg* 21:386–392, 1995.
21. Manche EE, Judge A, Maloney RK: Hyperopic lamellar keratoplasty. *Invest Ophthalmol Vis Sci* 36:S852, 1995.
22. Manche EE, Judge A, Maloney RK: Lamellar keratoplasty for hyperopia. *J Refract Surg* 12:42–49, 1996.
23. McDonald MB, Kaufman HE, Aquavella JV, Purrie DS, Hiles DA, Hunkeler JN, Keates RH Morgan KS, Sanders DR: The nationwide study of epikeratophakia for myopia. *Am J Ophthalmol* 103:375–383, 1987.
24. Moreira H, Campos M, Sawusch MR, McDonnell JM, McDonnell B, McDonnell PJ: Holmium laser thermokeratoplasty. *Ophthalmology* 100:752–761, 1993.
25. Newmann AC, McCarty GR: Hexagonal keratotomy for correction of low hyperopia: Preliminary results of a prospective study. *J Cataract Refract Surg* 14: 265–269, 1988.
26. Neumann AC, Sanders D, Raanan M, DeLuca M: Hyperopic thermokeratoplasty: clinical evaluation. *J Cataract Refract Surg* 17:830–838, 1991.
27. Seiler T, Matallana M, Bende T: Laser thermokeratoplasty by means of a pulsed holmium: YAG laser for hyperopic correction. *Refract Corneal Surg* 6:335–339, 1990.
28. Siganos DS, Siganos CS, Pallikaris IG: Clear lens extraction and intraocular lens implantation in normally sighted hyperopic eyes. *J Refract Corneal Surg* 10:117–124, 1994.
29. Worst JG, van der Veen G, Los LI: Refractive surgery for high myopia. The Worst-Fechner biconcave iris claw lens. *Doc Ophthalmol* 75:335–341, 1990.
30. Barraquer JI: Keratomileusis for myopia and aphakia. *Ophthalmology* 88(8):701–708, 1981.
31. Barraquer JI: Keratomileusis. *Int Surg* 48(2):103–117, 1967.

32. Barraquer C, Gutierrez AM, Espinosa A: Myopic keratomileusis: short term results. *Refract and Corneal Surg* 5(5):307–313, 1989.

33. Hollis S: Hyperopic lamellar keratoplasty. In Rozakis GW: *Refractive Lamellar Keratoplasty,* Thorofare, SLACK, 1994, pp. 77–78.

34. Binder PS, Zavala EY, Baumgartner SD, Nayak SK: Combined morphologic effects of cryolathing and lyophilisation on epikeratoplasty lenticules. *Arch Ophthalmol* 104:671–679, 1986.

35. Bohnke M, Draeger J, Klein L: Vacuum fixation of corneal lenticules for refractive surgery. In Draeger J, Winter R, eds. *New Microsurgical Concepts II. Cornea, Posterior Segment, External Microsurgery.* Basel, Karger, 1989, pp. 212–216.

36. Draeger J, Hackelbusch R. Experimentelle Untersuchungen und klinische Erfahrungen mit neuen Rotorinstrumenten. *Ophthalmol* 164:273–283, 1972.

37. Friedlander MH, Werblin TP, Kaufman HE, Granet NS: Clinical results of keratophakia and keratomileusis. *Ophthalmology* 88:716–720, 1981.

38. Hoffman NF, Harnisch JP: Effects of freezing on the corneal stroma of the rabbit after keratophakia. *Graefes Arch Clin Exp Ophthalmol* 215:243–248, 1981.

39. Hoffmann F, Jessen K: Keratokyphose zur optischen Korrektur der aphakie. *Fortschr Ophthalmol* 82:86–87, 1985.

40. Jessen K, Hoffmann F: Ein neues mikrokeratom zur lamellierenden refraktiven hornhautchirurgie. *Fortschr Ophthalmol* 82:88–90, 1985.

41. Jester JV, Logan DK, Verity SM: In vitro generation of chemotactic factors following keratorefractive surgery techniques in rabbit corneas. *Cornea* 2:69–80, 1983.

42. Swinger CA, Barraquer JI: Keratophakia and keratomileusis—clinical results. *Ophthalmology* 88:709–715, 1981.

43. Swinger CA, Krumeich J, Cassaday D: Planar lamellar refractive keratoplasty. *J Refract Surg* 2:17–22, 1986.

44. Hofmann RF, Bechara SJ: An independent evaluation of second generation suction microkeratomes. *Refract and Corneal Surg* 8(5):348–354, 1992.

45. Slade SG, Berkely RG: History of Keratomileusis. In Rozakis GW: *Refractive Lamellar Keratoplasty.* Thorofare, SLACK, 1994, pp. 1–16.

46. Poggio EC, Glynn RJ, Schein OD, Seddon JM, Shannon MJ, Scardino YA, Kenyon KR: The incidence of ulcerative keratitis among users of daily-wear and extended-wear soft contact lenses. *New Engl J Med* 321:779–783, 1989.

47. Altmann J, Grabner G, et al: Corneal lathing using the excimer laser and a computer-controlled positioning system: Part I—lathing of epikeratoplasty lenticules. *Refract Corneal Surg* 7(5):377–384, 1991.

48. Arenas-Archila E, Sanchez-Thorin JC, et al: Myopic keratomileusis in-situ: a preliminary report. *J Cataract Refract Surg* 17:424–435, 1991.

49. Bas AM, Nano HD: In situ myopic keratomileusis results in 30 eyes at 15 months. *Refract Corneal Surg* 7(3):223–231, 1991.

50. Buratto L, Ferrari M: Retrospective comparison of freeze and non-freeze myopic epikeratophakia. *Refract Corneal Surg* 5(2):94–97, 1989.

51. Carey BE: Synthetic keratophakia. In Brightbill FS, ed: *Corneal Surgery* 36:454–479, St. Louis/Washington, D.C., Mosby, 1986.

52. Colin J, Mimouni F, et al: The surgical treatment of high myopia: comparison of epikeratoplasty, keratomileusis and minus power anterior chamber lenses. *Refract Corneal Surg* 6(4):245–251, 1990.

53. Goosey JD, Prager TC, Goosey CB, Allison ME, Marvelli TL: Stability of refraction during two years after myopic epikeratoplasty. *Refract Corneal Surg* 6:4–8, 1990.

54. MacDonald MB: Epikeratophakia. In Brightbill FS, ed: *Corneal Surgery* 38:498–515, St. Louis/Washington, D.C., Mosby, 1986.

55. Maguire LJ, Klyce SD, Sawelson H, McDonald MB, Kaufman H: Visual distortion after myopic keratomileusis: computer analysis of keratoscopy photography. *Ophthal Surg* 18(5):352–356, 1987.

56. Nordan LT, Fallor MK: Myopic keratomileusis: 74 consecutive non-amblyopic cases with one year of follow-up. *J Refract Surg* 2(30):124–128, 1986.

57. Pallikaris IG, Papatzanaki ME, Siganos DS, Tsilimbaris MK: A corneal flap technique for laser in situ keratomileusis. *Arch Ophthalmol* 145:1699–1702, 1991.

58. Swinger CA, Barker BA: Prospective evaluation of myopic keratomileusis. *Ophthalmology* 91(7):785–792, 1984.

59. Wachtlin J, Schuler A, Hoffman F: Accuracy of corneal lenticules produced for lamellar refractive corneal surgery. *Cornea* 14(3):235–242, 1995.

60. Hoffman CJ, Rapuano CJ, Cohen EJ, Laibson PR: Displacement of corneal lenticule after automated lamellar keratoplasty. *Am J Ophthalmol* 118:109–111, 1994.

CHAPTER 13

Laser in Situ Keratomileusis (LASIK) for Hyperopia

Klaus Ditzen
Helda Huschka

INTRODUCTION

The history of keratomileusis goes back to the 1950s. Jose Ignacio Barraquer was the first to remove a layer of corneal tissue from the eye using an oscillating microkeratome.[1] The layer was frozen and then shaped to create a plus or minus lenticule in the 1980s proceeding from "freeze keratomileusis", which was beset by technical difficulties, Krumeich et al. developed "non freeze keratomileusis".[2] However, due to numerous technical problems this procedure also failed to become established. At the end of the 1980s, El Maghraby et al. developed keratomileusis "in situ", a procedure that enabled the refractive error to be corrected by intrasomal keratectomy.[3]

In a parallel development that was already under way by the early 1980s, excimer laser keratomileusis (photorefractive keratectomy or PRK) began to emerge. Initially, the excimer laser was tested on biological tissue.[4] The use of excimer lasers allowed the ablation of layers of corneal tissue only microns thick. Myopic PRK has been well established with excellent results. The use of PRK for hyperopia has been slower in development and has only recently been gathering researchers attention. The correction of hyperopia using PRK for hyperopic errors of less than 2.5 D seems to work well. Corrections of more than 2.5 diopters are more problematic. The most common postoperative complications are regression, severe haze, and increased glare sensitivity. The causes of these complications are assumed to be wound healing disorders, epithelial thickening and new collagen on the corneal surface.

LASIK

LASIK (laser in situ keratomileusis) is a procedure that combines a lamellar corneal flap and ablating the underlying cornea with an excimer laser. In this manner, it has eliminated some of the problems of poor predictability associated with keratomileusis and automated lamellar keratoplasty. High success rates in the correction of high myopia using LASIK were first reported by Buratto et al.,[5] Pallikaris et al.,[6,7] and Brint et al.[8] The corrections achieved were stable after one year and the interface also was still unscarred after 12 months.

Patients Selections and Preoperative Evaluation

In a 12-month period between September 1994 and September 1995, a total of 151 male and female patients of hyperopia. In the cases in which there was no explicit medical indication, the initial objective was a subjectively satisfactory correction with glasses or contact lenses.

A precondition of surgery was that the patient's refraction had been stable for at least 12 months. Exclusion criteria included unstable myopia, bullous keratopathy, rheumatic diseases, and collagenoses.

Contraindications

The absolute contraindications currently include corneal infections, collagen disorders (which are suspected of involving a risk of corneal ulceration), and corneal radius steeper than 7.2 mm. Prior to commencing therapy the patients were individually informed in detail, both verbally and in writing, of the nature, procedure, and risks of the operation. They confirmed their consent to the operation in writing.

Preoperative examinations included subjective and objective refraction, mesopic visual acuity (Rodenstock nyktometer), Keratometry (Javal and Zeiss keratometers), slit lamp examination, corneal mapping, and ultrasonic pacymetry.

Postoperatively, the patients were examined daily for one week and thereafter at intervals of 0, 5, 1, 2, 3, 6, and 12 months. The follow-up examinations routinely included measurement of visual acuity and refraction, slit lamp examination and keratometry. Mesopic visual acuity and corneal topography were checked after seven days, one month and six months.

CURRENT OPERATIVE TECHNIQUE

Like photorefractive keratectomy (PRK), the LASIK procedure involves modifying the radius of corneal curvature. To this end, a flap of superficial corneal layers can then be removed by photoablation with the excimer laser. The superficial layer of cornea is then folded back into position. Preoperatively the eye is locally anesthetized three times, each time with three drops of oxybarucain hydrochloride (4 mg/mL) at five-minute intervals. After inserting a lid retractor (Barraquer), the optic center of the cornea is identified with a marking instrument. The pneumatic fixation ring of microkeratome (Chiron) is then placed on the globe. The inner diameter of the corneal flap can be varied at will in a range between 4 and 9 mm, enabling different corneal flap areas to be chosen with the adjustable suction ring. (Fig. 13–1A). On the top of the suction ring there were two guides, intended to ensure that the microkeratome head cuts accurately. The microkeratome head consists of an oscillating knife, a motor and an interchangeable plate, the thickness of which determines the thickness of the flap to be resected. Fig. 13–1B For all the patients treated by us, a metal-plate with a layer thickness of 160 microns was used. In the cutting process, the microkeratome moves along the guides, incising the corneal surface with its oscillating blade. The corneal flap thus obtained consists of parts of the epithelium, Bowman's layer and the superficial stroma. The base of the flap is on the nasal side Fig. 13–1C. To prevent the corneal flap from being severed completely, a stop is fitted that automatically terminates the cutting procedure when a previously set distance has been covered. The flap is opened nasalward to expose the intrastromal ablation surface. Immediately prior to laser photoablation (MEL60, 193 nm argon fluoride excimer laser manufactured by Aesculap-Meditec, Heroldsberg,

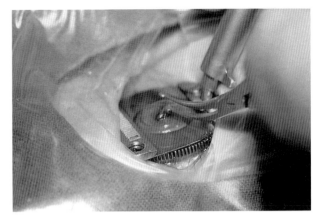

Fig. 13–1A Chiron keratome suction plate on eye with recently cut flap being lifted.

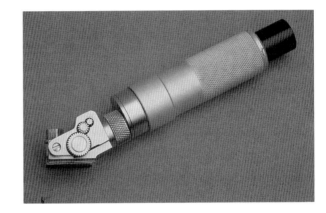

Fig. 13–1B Chiron Automated Corneal Shaper

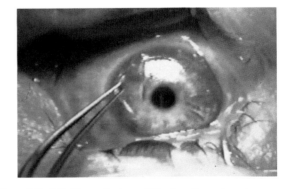

Fig. 13–1C Flap being lifted after keratome cut. (Courtesy of David Hardten M.D.).

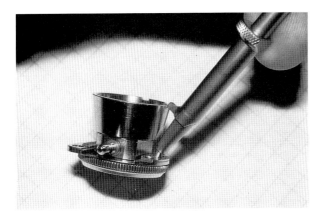

Fig. 13-2 Modified suction ring with adapter to hold Meditec handpiece and mask system.

Germany), the eye was once again fixed with a suction ring and the centration of the eye checked with a marking instrument. With a special suction ring (Fig. 13-2) various handpieces can be fixed to the eye. (Fig. 13-3) Depending on the refractive error, masks with differently shaped aperture patterns are used, through which the laser beam strikes the stroma as it sweeps back and forth. The openings in the hyperopia mask are peripheral, resulting in a peripheral ablation and central steepening. In contrast, the myopia mask has an hourglass-shaped central opening which produces a central flattening of the cornea. Both masks rotate through 360°, with adjustable speeds (angular increments). After each sweep of the laser beam the rotation mask moves by one angular increment.

After completion of the laser procedure and removal of the suction ring, the surface is flushed with balanced saline and the corneal flap is laid back over the treated region of the stroma. One drop each of homatropine, gentamicin and Ketorolac solution (Acular) are administered immediately after the operation. From the first postoperative day onward, one drop of gentamicin is given three times a day for five days. One week postoperatively this regime is replaced with one drop of Fluorometholone 0.1% three times a day. This therapy is maintained for four weeks. The dosage is then reduced to one drop a day for one month, after which treatment is terminated.

Results

In a 12 month period from September 1994 to September 1995, a total of 43 eyes (43 patients) underwent LASIK for hyperopia. Depending on the preoperative refraction, each eye was assigned to one of two refraction groups. The resulting distribution in the individual groups was as follows: 20 eyes from +0.00 to +4.00D in Group I, with a mean patient age of 42 years (range, 22 to 72 years); 23 eyes from +4.25 to +9.00D in Group II, with a mean patient age of 37 years (range, 24 to 45 years). See Table 13-1.

Postoperative Refraction

In both groups, emmetropia was aimed for. Uncorrected visual acuity in the first week postoperatively fluctuated by 1–2 Snellen lines in 98% of the patients. Therefore it was stable in all patients. Complications, which are discussed below, occurred in 2% of the patients.

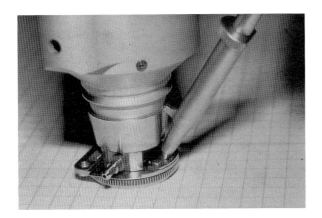

Fig. 13-3 MEL 60 handpiece attached to adapter and suction plate.

Table 13-1. Hyperopic Groups

Hyperopia groups	Mean age, (Range), years	Preop. sph. (D)	Number of cases
I	42.35 (22–72)	+1.0 to +4.0	20
II	36.78 (24–45)	+4.25 to +9.0	23

HYPEROPIA

Group I (20 patients with +0 to +4.0D): The mean spherical equivalent decreased from 2.05 +/ −1.70 D preoperatively to 0.26 +/−0.95 at one month and to +0.33D +/−1.32 D at one year. (*See* Fig. 13–4)

Group II (23 patients with +4.25D): The mean spherical equivalent decreased from +5.28 +/ −1.92 D preop to 1.03 +/−1.40 D at one month to 1.91 +/−1.83 D at one year (*See* Fig. 13–5)

Best Corrected Visual Acuity

In 20 eyes (46.5%) no change in visual acuity was observed postoperatively (from average of 20/60). Six patients (14%) had gained one Snellen line (from an average of 20/40 to 20/32). Five eyes (11.6%) gained two lines (on average from 20/30 to 20/25, and four eyes (9.3%) more than three lines (on average from 20/50 to 20/25). *See* Table 13–2

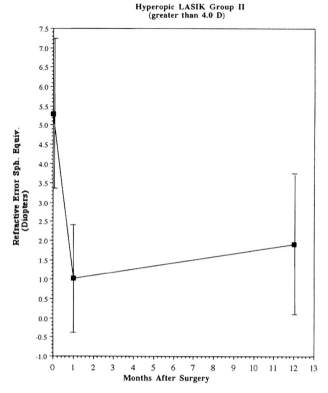

Fig. 13–5 Change in spherical equivalent over time. Group II (hyperopia, 23 patients with >+4.0D).

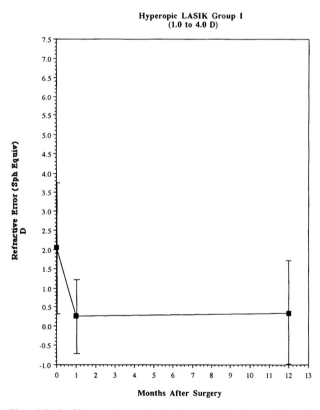

Fig. 13–4 Change in spherical equivalent over time in Group I (hyperopia, 20 patients with 0 to 3.75 D).

Table 13–2. Lost and Gain of Best Corrected and Uncorrected Visual Acuity after Hyperopic LASIK

Group	Best Corrected Spectacle VA	Uncorrected visual acuity
3 or more lines lost	6.0%	0%
2 lines lost	4.6%	0%
1 line lost	6.9%	2.3%
No change	46.5%	16.2%
1 line gained	14%	14%
2 lines gained	11.6%	25%
3 or more lines gained	9.3%	41.4%

A loss of one Snellen line (on average from 20/21 to 20/36) occurred in three patients' eyes (6.9%); of two lines (from 20/22 to 20/28) in three patients (6%), and of three lines (from 20/29 to 20/34) in two eyes (4.6%).

Uncorrected Visual Acuity

The results are also summarized in Table 2. In seven eyes (16.2%) there was no postoperative change in visual acuity (from 20/200). Six eyes (14%) gained one Snellen line (from 20/200 to 20/100), and in 11 patients (25%) a gain of two lines was achieved (from 20/90 to 20/46). Eighteen eyes (41.4%) showed an improvement of three or more lines (20/100 to 20/30). Visual acuity deteriorated only in one patient (2.2), from 20/66 to 20/100.

Complications

Based on the results in the treated cases presented here, the following complications were observed in the course of follow up over a 12 month period. These are summarized in Table 13–3.

Epithelial Ingrowth
Six cases of epithelial ingrowth (14%) were seen. This represents growth of epithelial cells into the interface that results form incising the cornea. After the resected corneal layer (i.e., the flap) is put back in place, there is a risk that while the wound is healing, epithelial cells will grow into the surgical incision, i.e., at the wound margins. Since, under physiological conditions, the 8mm-diameter ablation

zone which we opted for is larger than the maximum pupillary diameter, the epithelial invasion probably did not affect the optical axis. In most cases, the patients did not complain of any reduction in quality of vision such as glare or contrast sensitivity, even though the epithelial cells reached the optic axis. This necessitates lifting the corneal flap and scraping off the epithelial cells from the back of the flap and the bed.

Haze
In the LASIK procedure, postoperative epithelial scarring (haze), which occurs relatively frequently in PRK, can be almost completely avoided by leaving the epithelium and Bowman's layer untouched. In four cases, Grade 1–2 haze nevertheless developed following therapy but cleared up within six months.

Decentration
One difficulty during surgery is the risk of eccentric ablation. By using a suction ring and a marking instrument, it can be reduced or minimized. Eccentric ablation occurred in two patients, whereas astigmatism showed minimal changes in three patients.

Irregular Astigmatism
Unevenness of the ablated surface is characterized by temporary impairments of visual acuity. It presumably occurs as a result of irregular cutting by the keratome knife or micro-deformations in the corneal structures. Two patients (1%) were affected.

Glare
Daylight glare sensitivity (so called white haze) was reported by one patient only. It resolved within three months. Seven patients confirmed when explicitly asked that they were sensitive to glare in darkness and at twilight. There was no functional impairment.

Other Complications
Prophylactic postoperative topical steroid treatment can sometimes lead to increases in intraocular pressure. We have not yet seen any occurrences of this or of other possible complications such as corneal inflammation, ptosis, diplopia or anisometropia.

Table 13–3. Postoperative Complications

Complications	No. of cases
Epithelial invasion	6 (14%)
Haze	4 (9%)
Decentration	2 (5%)
Central islands	2 (5%)
Glare sensitivity	1 (1%)
Diplopia	0
Anisometropia	0
Steroid-induced increase in IOP	0

DISCUSSION

With the LASIK-procedure it was possible to treat hyperopic refractive errors of more than three diopters with less regression, a better predictability, and a more stable refraction.

In this one year-report there were 43 hyperopic eyes, divided in two groups (1 to 4 diopters and 4.5 to 9 diopters). Regression in group I was +0.75 diopters, and in group II it was 2.5 diopters. The predictability to within one diopter in the scattergram were 95% in group I and 75% in group II. It was much better in comparison to hyperopic PRK, using the same 7.5 mm iris mask. The hyperopic treatment profile was a 4 mm untreated central zone, a 1.5 mm steepening transition zone and a 2 mm excavated refractive ring zone. The complications of the procedure most often involved the flap. Complications included flap dislocation and irregular astigmatism, especially in the higher hyperopic refractive errors. A flap diameter of more than 8.5 mm would be superior to ablate a larger refractive zone to correct hyperopic refractive errors more than +8 diopters.

SUMMARY

The LASIK procedure is a two step procedure. First, there is a microkeratome cut followed by an excimer laser ablation. In 43 hyperopic eyes, the results in hyperopic errors of more than 4 diopters were encouraging. There was lower regression, minimal haze and a better stability of the refraction.

REFERENCES

1. Barraquer JL: Method for cutting lamellar grafts: new orientation for refractive surgery. *Ophthalmol Zh* 261–271, 1985.
2. Krumeich JH: Indications, techniques and complications of myopic keratomileusis. *Int Ophthalmol Clin* 23:75–92, 1983.
3. El-Maghraby MA, Vitero E, Ruiz L: Keratomileusis in situ to correct high myopia. *Ophthalmology* 95, 272–281, 1988.
4. Trokel SL, Srinivasan R, Braren B: Excimer laser surgery of the cornea. *Am J Ophthalmol* 96:710–715, 1983.
5. Buratto L, Ferrart M, Genisi C: Myopic keratomileusis with the excimer laser. *Refract Corneal Surg* 9(1): 12–19, 1993.
6. Pallikaris IG, Papatzanaki ME, Stathi EZ: Lader in situ keratomileusis. *Laser Surg Med* 10 (5):463–468, 1990.
7. Faschinger C, Faulborn J, Ganser K: Infectious corneal ulcers once with endophthalmitis after photorefractive keratectomy with disposable contact lens. *Klin Monatsbl Augenheilk* 206:96–102, 1995.
8. Brint S, Ostrick M, Fischer C: Six months' results of the multicenter phase I study of excimer laser myopic keratomileusis. *J Cataract Refract Surg* 20 (6):610–615, 1994.

section V

Intrastromal Procedures

A. Non-Contact

Intrastromal Procedures: the Use of the Noncontact Holmium:YAG Laser for Correction of Hyperopia—Sunrise Technologies Experience

Douglas D. Koch
Rogelio Villarreal V
Thomas Kohnen
Peter J. McDonnell
Paolo Vinciguerra
Richard Menefee
Michael Berry

INTRODUCTION

Thermal keratoplasty (heat-generated corneal shaping) has a long, but mostly disappointing, history,[1] beginning with Lans' classic cautery experiments in 1898[2] and extending to modern preclinical and clinical laser thermal keratoplasty (LTK) studies,[1,3-38] in which laser light has been used to produce corneal heating and shaping. The "Holy Grail" of thermal keratoplasty has always been to achieve safe, effective, predictable, and stable corneal shaping, but almost all thermal keratoplasty quests have been plagued by regression of induced refractive correction.

This chapter summarizes clinical results for correction of simple hyperopia obtained by noncontact holmium:yttrium aluminum garnet (Ho:YAG) LTK using the Sunrise Technologies Corneal Shaping System (CSS). In contrast to other thermal keratoplasty devices and procedures, the Sunrise CSS experience is that stable corrections of low hyperopia can be achieved without complications such as induced irregular astigmatism.

CLINICAL HISTORY

Five controlled clinical studies using the Sunrise Corneal Shaping System (CSS) have been completed.[32-34,36-39] Aspects of these studies are summarized in Table 14–1. LTK treatment parameters were initially explored by *in vitro* experiments on animal and human eyebank eyes[1,17,20,25,27-28] and by a basic safety study on poorly sighted eyes[32] (Study 1—U.S. Phase I in Table 1). The first Sunrise CSS clinical study on sighted eyes (in Monterrey, Mexico)[33] (Study 2—MTY1 in Table 1) used now obsolete LTK treatment parameters including 10 pulses of Ho:YAG laser light delivered simultaneously into 8 treatment spots arranged in a symmetrical octagonal array on a 6 mm centerline diameter ring (Group 2—Figs. 14–1 and 14–2). The first U.S. study on sighted eyes[34,36-37] (Study 3—U.S. Phase IIa in Table 1) used similar treatment parameters for one group of patients (one-ring [3A]), but added a "skewed" two-ring treatment pattern (with spots rotated 22.5° between rings) for a second group of patients (Group 3B—Figs. 1 and 2), with centrifugal (inner, followed by outer) ring treatments. Both of these clinical studies used fixed treatment geometries and varied treatment pulse energies to "titrate" the amounts of refractive corrections produced by one-ring and two-ring treatment patterns. A second international clinical study on sighted eyes in Monterrey[38] (Study 4—MTY2 in Table 1) used a fixed treatment pulse energy and two centrifugal (inner, followed by outer) rings with all spots on radials, varying ring diameters to "titrate" refractive corrections (e.g., Group 4A—Figs. 14–1 and 14–2).

Table 14–1. Sunrise Corneal Shaping System Clinical Studies.

Study #—Title	n	Patients* nm/nf	Age (y)	LTK Treatment Parameters** D (mm)	N	M	Ep (mJ)	ΔUDVA	1-Year-Post-Operative Results*** ΔSE (D)	ΔCyl (D)	Stability	Ref(s)
1—U.S. Phase I	10	5/5	61 ± 15	≤ 6	≤ 32	≤ 10	≤ 230	n/a	n/a	n/a	n/a	32
2—MTY1	17	5/12	55 ± 7	6	8	10	159 to 199	0.14—0.39	−0.79 ± 0.65	0.16 ± 0.49	0.59	33
3—U.S. Phase IIa												34,
Group 3A	20	5/15	55 ± 8	6	8	10	208 to 242	0.30—0.60	−0.55 ± 0.33	0.25 ± 0.29	0.54	36–37
Group 3B	8	2/6	55 ± 8	6/7S	8/8	10/10	224 to 240	0.15—0.43	−1.64 ± 0.61	0.47 ± 0.53	0.43	
4—MTY2												38
Group 4A	12	3/9	57 ± 5	5/6	8/8	5/5	240	0.12—0.27	−2.08 ± 1.13	−0.92 ± 1.46	0.80	
Group 4B	6	1/5	50 ± 14	6/7	8/8	5/5	240	0.10—0.49	−1.83 ± 0.88	−0.17 ± 0.38	0.62	
Group 4C	21	5/16	63 ± 11	6.5/7.5	8/8	5/5	240	0.10—0.36	−1.22 ± 0.88	0.15 ± 0.58	0.46	
5—MZA												39
Group 5A	8	6/2	42 ± 10	6/7/8	8/8/8	7/7/7	240	0.19—0.55	−2.15 ± 1.6	ca. 0.15	ca. 0.43	
Group 5B	8	6/2	42 ± 10	6/7S/8	8/8/8	7/7/7	240	0.17—0.43	−1.50 ± 1.6	ca. 0.15	ca. 0.30	

*n—Total number of patient eyes, n_m/n_f—Number of male/female patient eyes, Age — Mean − standard deviation (SD)

**D—Centerline ring diameter(s), S—Skewed spots, N—Number(s) of spots, M—Number(s) of pulses, E_p—Pulse energy

***ΔUDVA—Change in Uncorrected Distance Visual Acuity (decimal units, pre − post, geometric means except for Study 5—MZA),

ΔSE—Change in Spherical Equivalent [Subjective Manifest Refraction (SMR), post-minus pre-, mean ± SD],

ΔCyl—Change in Cylinder (SMR, post- minus pre-, plus cylinder convention, mean ± SD),

Stability—Ratio of mean Delta SE values for 1 week post- divided by 1 year post-,

n/a—not applicable (safety study only)

136

Hyperopia Correction Treatment Patterns

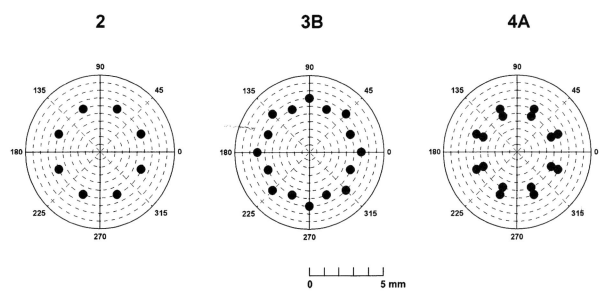

Fig. 14–1. Hyperopia correction treatment patterns for Clinical Studies 2, 3B, and 4A—*see* Table 14–1.

Another international clinical study by Vinciguerra, et al. (in Monza, Italy)[39] (Study 5—MZA in Table 1) explored the relative merits of "skewed" spots vs. radial spots in three-ring bilateral treatments applied centrifugally (inner, followed by middle, followed by outer rings). Since all outcomes (amount of refractive correction, size and regularity of the central steepened zone, patient satisfaction, etc.) proved that the radial pattern is superior, "skewed" spot treatments have now been abandoned for hyperopia correction. ("Skewed" spot treatments may, however, be useful to produce multifocal corneas that are potentially useful for presbyopia correction.) Ten-pulse treatments have also been abandoned, due to the results of histology studies[35,40] and to superior clinical results obtained with 5-pulse[38] and 7-pulse[41] treatments.

All the above clinical studies have been completed using a centrifugal (inner to outer) sequence of treatment rings when 2 or more rings of laser spots are delivered. An additional international clinical study by Vinciguerra, et al. in Monza, Italy (personal communication) is exploring the relative merits of a centripetal (outer to inner) sequence of

treatment rings compared to the original centrifugal sequence. In many cases, the centripetal sequence may be better.

At present, the Sunrise Corneal Shaping System is in use at over 40 clinics worldwide. Much anecdotal information is available from these clinics, but the present chapter discusses only the results of controlled clinical studies that have well-defined protocols and long-term follow-up results on large percentages of the treated patient eyes.

CURRENT TECHNIQUE

The current Sunrise noncontact Ho:YAG LTK procedure uses a "minimalist approach" toward thermal modification of intrastromal collagen. Minimal intervention with a minimum amount of laser energy is used to thermally modify a sufficient volume of intrastromal collagen[33] without causing significant long-term biological, biochemical, and/or biomechanical responses of the cornea to thermal injury. Histological studies (including immunohistochemical analyses of procollagen and proteo-

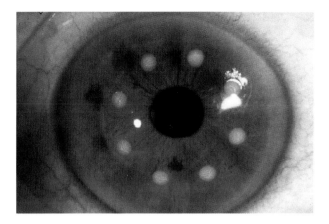

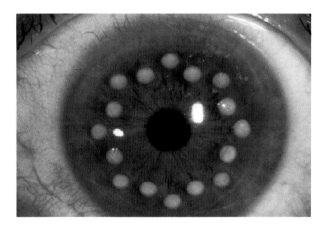

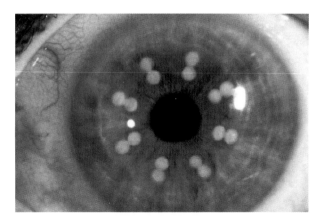

Fig. 14–2. Slit-lamp photographs of corneas approximately 1 week after treatment for patients in Clinical Studies 2 (top), 3B (middle), and 4A (bottom)—*see* Table 14–1.

glycan syntheses accompanying wound healing response),[35,40] together with clinical studies on regression in patient treatment groups, are being used to develop improved treatment algorithms that yield effective and stable refractive corrections.

The Sunrise Corneal Shaping System (CSS) simultaneously projects "beamlets" of Ho:YAG laser light (wavelength: 2.13 μm, pulse duration: 250 μs full width at half maximum intensity, pulse repetition frequency: 5 Hz) in a noncontact mode (through a modified slit-lamp biomicroscope) onto a maximum of eight treatment spots on the cornea. Each beamlet has equivalent energy to yield a symmetrical treatment within each ring of spots (Figures 14–1 and 14–2). Rings are applied individually, requiring multiple centrations for multiple rings to assure accurate inter-ring concentricity and angular orientation (*e.g.*, spots on symmetrical radials as in Group 4A—Figs. 14–1 and 14–2). Ring diameters and angular orientations are adjusted manually. The number and energies of treatment pulses are set by the physician using a microprocessor-based controller.

The current treatment protocol includes administration of topical anaesthetic drops (0.5% proparacaine solution—Alcaine™, Alcon Laboratories, Fort Worth, TX) beginning at least 30 minutes prior to treatment, with one drop at 5 minute intervals up to a total of 4 drops. A lid speculum is introduced 5 minutes after the last proparacaine drop is administered, and the eyelids are held open 3 minutes to allow the tear film to dry before treatment. (Some clinics use forced air drying to obtain faster, more thorough drying.) The timing of proparacaine drops and tear film drying is designed to standardize epithelial swelling[42] and corneal hydration; both of these factors affect the penetration of Ho:YAG laser light into the corneal stroma where collagen modification occurs.

The patient sits facing the CSS slit-lamp delivery system and views a fixation light while the physician views the eye through the slit-lamp biomicroscope. The ideal treatment involves: 1) centration of the eight laser beam spots with respect to the pupillary center and along the line-of-sight[43], 2) focussing of each treatment spot on the surface of the cornea, and 3) motionless delivery during the 1- to 1.4-second treatment (corresponding to 5 to 7 laser pulses delivered at 5 Hz). The physician obtains centration by centering red helium neon (HeNe, wavelength: 633 nm) laser tracer beams around the entrance pupil while the patient views a red light emitting diode (LED) fixation source. Calibrated green HeNe (wavelength: 543 nm) laser focussing aid beams are used to focus treatment Ho:YAG laser beams on the surface of the cornea. The patient is advised to remain motionless during the treatment. (In some clinics, patients practice the procedure prior to treatment.) The physician uses the slit-lamp joy stick to adjust centration and focussing and then steps on a foot pedal to deliver Ho:YAG laser light using the predetermined treatment pattern, pulse number, and pulse energy. Typically, the patient does not feel the actual laser energy delivery. Multiple rings are delivered in one sitting by repeating centration and focussing steps, taking care to obtain concentric, symmetrical multiple ring treatment patterns (e.g., Groups 3B and 4A in Figures 1 and 2).

Post-operatively, antibiotic solution (either 0.3% tobramycin—Tobrex™; Alcon Laboratories, Fort Worth, TX or 0.3% norfloxacin—Noroxin™; Merck, Sharp and Dohme, Cedex, France) and diclofenac sodium—Voltaren™ (CibaVision Ophthalmics, Duluth, GA) are prescribed for administration to the treated eye four times daily until the epithelium heals (typically, within three days). The patient is instructed to take 1 or 2 analgesic tablets (plain acetaminophen or acetaminophen with codeine—Tylenol#3™) every 4 hours as needed for pain management. No corticosteroids are used.

Visual rehabilitation is immediate (leading some clinics to perform bilateral treatments in one sitting), with no requirement for a contact lens and/or eyepatch. Until the epithelium heals, the patient may experience some discomfort (pain, foreign body sensation, tearing, photophobia, etc.), which is reduced by the current 5- to 7-pulse, compared to the original 10-pulse, treatment regimen.

Previously, treatment algorithms were based on short-term (e.g., 30 day postoperative) clinical data. Currently, the availability of treatment algorithms that produce more effective and more stable refractive corrections[38] permit treatments based on the intended change at 6 months or 1 year postoperatively. Regression of the initial overcorrection (from, for example, −1 D immediately after treatment to −0.5 D at six months postoperatively) is now very acceptable to the patient.

RESULTS

This section is organized according to requirements stipulated by the U.S. Food and Drug Administration (FDA) to demonstrate that a laser refractive surgery device is safe and effective.[44] These FDA requirements are the "gold standard" in the U.S. to achieve pre-market approval (PMA), as well as internationally to achieve acceptance by both non-U.S. regulatory agencies and physicians. FDA requirements[44] and current Sunrise Corneal Shaping System (CSS) achievements toward those requirements are summarized in Table 14–2.

Safety

In order to be considered safe by the FDA, a candidate laser refractive surgery device and procedure must meet three prinicipal clinical safety criteria (in addition to engineering/technical criteria for device electrical safety, etc.); these are indicated as FDA Requirements S1 through S3 in Table 14–2. The Sunrise CSS has met or exceeded all of these requirements in controlled clinical studies to date. In addition to the worldwide clinical experience is that there are no safety concerns for the Sunrise noncontact Ho:YAG LTK procedure. The worst case scenario (obtained in some early treatments using now-obsolete 10-pulse algorithms) is that the patient does not obtain improved vision due to inadequate initial treatment and/or to regression of initial effect.

Effectiveness

In order to be considered effective by the FDA, a candidate laser refractive surgery device and procedure must meet two principal clinical effectiveness criteria (in addition to engineering/technical criteria for device effectiveness); these are indicated as FDA Requirements E1 and E2 (together with an optional Requirement E3) in Table 14–2.

Requirement E1 (predictability of the intended refractive correction) has not yet been demonstrated using current treatment algorithms; however, if the actual mean 1-year postoperative Delta SE, SMR values for Clinical Study 4 (MTY2—see Table 14–1)[38] are used as predictor values for intended Delta SEs, the three treatment group results exceeded FDA requirements. Demonstra-

Table 14–2. Comparison of FDA Requirements and Sunrise Corneal Shaping System (CSS) Results.

FDA Requirement	Time Post-	Sunrise CSS Results	Comments	Ref(s)
S1: ≤5.0% loss of ≥ 2 lines of BSCDVA in treated eyes	≥ 6 m	0.0% loss of ≥ 2 lines of BSCDVA	Sunrise noncontact LTK induces little or no irregular astigmatism and does not produce corneal haze in the central visual zone	33–34, 37–39
S2: ≤ 1.0% nonsight-threatening Adverse Events (AEs); nonexistent or rare sight-threatening AEs	All	0.0% incidence	The only complications are those anticipated for short-term epithelial damage	33–34, 37–39
S3: ≤10.0% loss of central corneal endothelial cell density (ECD) in a cohort of treated eyes	≥ 6 m	At 1 y, 0.4% loss in a cohort of 12 treated eyes	At 1 y, 0.7% loss in fellow (untreated) eyes	34, 37
E1: ≥ 75% of treated eyes are within ± 1.0 D and ≥ 50% are within ± 0.5 D of the attempted refractive change	6 m	88% within ± 1.0 D and 71% within ±0.5 D	Study 4 (MTY2) only; actual means of Delta SE, SMR values used as predictors of attempted Delta SEs	38
E2: ≥ 95% of treated eyes are within ± 1.0 D and 6 m refraction	12 m	97% within ± 1.0 D	Study 4 (MTY2) only	38
E3(optional?): ≥ 90% of treated eyes have UDVA of 20/40 or better and ≥ 50% have UDVA of 202/20 or better	6 m	Not yet tested	Initial treatment algorithms did not account for long-term regression	

S—Safety, E—Effectiveness, BSCDVA—Best Spectacle-Corrected Distance Visual Acuity, UDVA—Uncorrected Distance Visual Acuity, m—month; compiled from Ref. 44

tion of this predictability requirement must still be achieved in future phases of the U.S. Clinical Trial.

Requirement E2 (stability of the intended refractive correction) has been demonstrated in all three treatment groups of Clinical Study 4 (MTY2—see Table 1).[38] Requirement E3 for uncorrected distance visual acuity (UDVA) outcomes, must still be achieved in future phases of the U.S. Clinical Trial. At present, however, large improvements in UDVA have been achieved (see Table 1). In Clinical Study 4 (MTY2),[38] most of the patients (94% or 28 of 30 with 1-year follow-up examinations) had improvements in UDVA and 13 of 30 (43%) had UDVA of 0.5 (Snellen: 20/40) or better; the average improvement was more than 3.5 lines of Snellen visual acuity. As an added benefit, pre-existing astigmatism was reduced significantly for Groups 4A and 4B (see Table 14–1), the smaller diameter treatment groups. It is likely that the new treatment algorithms developed in Clinical Study 4 will successfully treat patients with 1 to 2 D of hyperopia.

The current 5-pulse treatment algorithms developed in Clinical Study 4 (MTY2—see Table 14–1)[38] represent a major advance over earlier (now obsolete) 10-pulse treatment algorithms. The time courses of mean changes in spherical equivalents (Delta SE, SMR) for Clinical Studies 2, 3B, and 4A (matching treatment patterns in Figs. 14–1 and 14–2) are shown in Fig. 14–3. The current refractive corrections obtained in Clinical Study 4A (using a two-ring treatment pattern at 5/6mm ring diameters with 5 pulses of laser light) have much greater stability than earlier refractive corrections.

Progress in obtaining larger and more stable hyperopia corrections is summarized in Fig. 14–4, which shows values of Delta SE and Stability (defined in Table 14–1) for each Sunrise CSS clinical study at 1 year postoperative examinations. The largest need for hyperopia correction in mature adults (≥45 years old) is low hyperopia of +1.0 to + 3.0 D (SE)[45]; the LTK treatment algorithm used for Clinical Study 4A already provides high stability

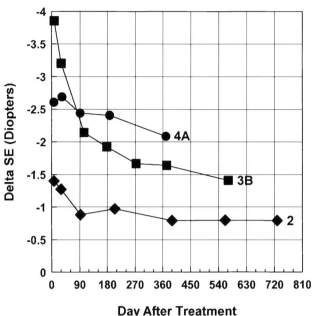

Fig. 14–3. Means of the changes in spherical equivalents of subjective manifest refraction measurements as a function of mean days after treatment for Clinical Studies 2, 3B, and 4A—see Table 14–1.

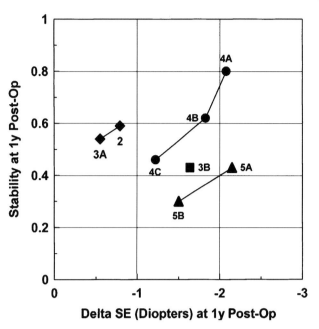

Fig. 14–4. 1-Year postoperative effectiveness (Delta SE) and stability (defined in Table 14–1) for clinical studies on sighted eyes listed in Table 14–1.

(*ca.* 0.8) corrections at the +2.1 D level, but further extensions are required to treat patients with greater amounts of hyperopia.

COMPLICATIONS

Sunrise noncontact Ho:YAG LTK treatments are free from unanticipated complications (i.e., non-transient adverse events). In four controlled clinical studies on sighted patients (*see* Table 14–1), there have been no adverse events. In the earliest clinical studies (Studies 2 and 3, *see* Table 1),[33–34,37] patient and/or physician motion during treatment occasionally led to ineffective treatments. However, improvements in technique, as well as the reduced number of laser pulses and reduced treatment time of current algorithms, have reduced the motion problem. Centration has not been a problem; the mean decentration in the first clinical study[33] was less than 0.5 mm and even extreme decentrations up to

1.25 mm did not appear to induce astigmatism. Using current techniques, experienced physicians have no significant decentration errors; in addition, the mean induced refractive astigmatism is typically less than 0.5 D within the first two weeks after treatment, drops to less than 0.25 D at 3 months, and exhibits a net decrease at 6 months and longer.[38]

Treatment spots (*ca.* 0.6 mm diameter) are initially opacified; opacification is probably due to a combination of stromal collagen modification and stromal hydration change, both of which produce light scattering sites in the treated volumes. Opacifications gradually fade so that they are barely visible under normal room lights a few months after treatment. Glare and contrast sensitivity testing indicate that peripheral corneal opacities produced by LTK do not degrade vision.[33–34,37] This result is understandable since the peripheral opacities are outside pupillary diameters of typical patients (≥45 years old, *see* Table 1) under both photopic and scotopic vision conditions. For smaller diameter treatments (e.g., Treatment Pattern 4A in Figs. 14–1 and 14–2), it is still necessary to perform night vision testing[46] to assure that opacities extending into the paracentral corneal zone do not compromise night vision.

FUTURE PLANS AND DEVELOPMENTS

New Sunrise CSS clinical studies are directed toward the following goals:

1. Extension of the range of hyperopia correction to patients with preoperative SEs of +3.0 D and larger,
2. Development of refined treatment algorithms with improved long-term stability,
3. Extension of treatments to younger (<40 year old) patients, who appear to receive reduced refractive corrections compared to older patients,[41]
4. Development of enhancement treatment/staged treatment protocols to reduce outcome variability,
5. Development of treatment algorithms for overcorrected postphotorefractive keratectomy (post-PRK) patients, who appear to obtain larger LTK effects than patients with no previous corneal surgery,[41]
6. Development of treatment algorithms for post-radial keratotomy (post-RK) patients who have experienced progressive hyperopic shift (PHS) following RK,
7. Development of treatment algorithms for presbyopic patients—simple monovision may be prescribed, but since LTK treatment (particularly with a "skewed" geometry of multiple rings) leads to increased corneal asphericity,[36] there is a potentiality for tailoring multifocal corneas to patient needs,
8. Development of new technology for improved treatments (*e.g.*, reduction of initial epithelial damage so that treatments are purely intrastromal), and
9. Development of treatment protocols and algorithms for correction of astigmatism (including iatrogenic astigmatism).

It is worth noting that, after nearly a century of previous attempts to use heat to change corneal shape, the Sunrise noncontact Ho:YAG LTK procedure has finally produced refractive corrections with long-term stability. We believe that this procedure, still in its infancy, has great promise to become the method of choice for the correction of low hyperopia and presbyopia.

ACKNOWLEDGMENTS

The authors thank the sponsors of this study and gratefully acknowledge JoLene Carranza, COT, Jenny Garbus, BS, and Carol Kim, BA for administrative and clinical assistance, Theresa Nazaroff, MA for regulatory advice, and Giorgio Dorin, BS(PI in Italy) and Bruce Sand, MD for clinical advice and encouragement.

This work was supported, in part, by an unrestricted grant from Research to Prevent Blindness, Inc., New York, NY, by Deutsche Forschungsgemeinschaft (DFG) Postdoctoral Research Grants Ko 1595/1-1 and 1-2, and by core grant EY03040 from the National Eye Institute, Bethesda, MD.

Reprint requests should be addressed to: Douglas D. Koch, MD, Cullen Eye Institute, Baylor College of Medicine, 6501 Fannin, NC-200, Houston, TX 77030-3498. Telephone: (713) 798-6443. FAX: (713) 798-3027. E-mail: DDKMD@aol.com

REFERENCES

1. Koch DD, Berry MJ, Vassiliadis AJ, Haft EA: Noncontact holmium:YAG laser thermal keratoplasty. In Salz JJ, ed: *Corneal Laser Surgery*. St. Louis, MO, Mosby-Year Book, 1995, pp247–254.
2. Lans LJ. Experimentelle Untersuchungen über die Entstehung von Astigmatismus durch nicht-perforierende Corneawunden. *Graefes Arch Clin Exp Ophthalmol* 45:117–152, 1898.
3. Peyman GA, Larson B, Raichand M, Andrews AH: Modification of rabbit corneal curvature with use of carbon dioxide laser burns. *Ophthalmic Surg* 11: 325–329, 1980.
4. Kanoda AN, Sorokin AS. Laser correction of hypermetropic refraction. In Fyodorov SN, ed: *Microsurgery of the Eye: Main Aspects*. Moscow, MIR Publishers, 1987, pp147–154.

5. Householder J, Horwitz LS, Lowe KW, Murrillo A: Laser-induced thermal keratoplasty. *Proc SPIE* 1066: 18–23, 1989.

6. Seiler T, Matallana M, Bende T. Laser thermokeratoplasty by means of a pulsed holmium:YAG laser for hyperopic correction. *Refract Corneal Surg* 6:328–333, 1990.

7. Spears KG, Horn G, Serafin J. Corneal refractive correction by laser thermal keratoplasty. *Proc SPIE* 1202:334–340, 1990.

8. Horn G, Spears KG, Lopez O, Lewicky A, Yang X, Riaz M, Wang R, Silva D, Serafin J: New refractive method for laser thermal keratoplasty with the Co:MgF$_2$ laser. *J Cataract Refract Surg* 16:611–616, 1990.

9. Valderrama GL, Fredin LG, Berry MJ, Harpole GM, Demsey BP: Temperature distributions in laser-irradiated tissues. *Proc SPIE* 1427:200–213, 1991.

10. Koch DD, Padrick TD, Halligan DT, Krenee BD, Menefee RF, Berry MJ, Rocha M, Sperling HG: HF chemical laser photothermal keratoplasty. *Invest Ophthalmol Vis Sci* 32:994, 1991.

11. Bende T, Seiler T, Matallana T: Regression of hyperopic correction with the Ho:YAG laser is dependent on coagulation depth. *Invest Ophthalmol Vis Sci* 32: 995, 1991.

12. Zhou Z, Ren Q, Simon G, Parel J: Thermal modeling of laser photothermokeratoplasty (LPTK). *Proc SPIE* 1644:61–71, 1992.

13. Durrie DS, Seiler T, King MC, Muller DF, Sacharoff AC: Application of the holmium:YAG laser for refractive surgery. *Proc SPIE* 1644:56–60, 1992.

14. Chandonnet A, Bazin R, Sirois C, Belanger PA: CO$_2$ laser annular thermokeratoplasty: a preliminary study. *Lasers Surg Med* 12:264–273, 1992.

15. Koch DD, Padrick TD, Menefee RF, Berry MJ, Sperling HG: Laser photothermal keratoplasty: nonhuman primate results. *Invest Ophthalmol Vis Sci* 33: 768, 1992.

16. Seiler T: Ho:YAG laser thermokeratoplasty for hyperopia. *Ophthalmol Clinics North Am* 5:773–780, 1992.

17. Koch DD, Abarca A, Menefee RF, Berry MJ: Ho:YAG laser thermal keratoplasty: *in vitro* experiments. *Invest Ophthalmol Vis Sci* 34:1246, 1993.

18. King MC, Muller DF, Sacharoff AC, Seiler T, Durrie DS: Application of the Ho:YAG laser for refractive surgery: an update of clinical progress. *Proc SPIE* 1877:52–56, 1993.

19. Ren Q, Melgar TM, Parel JM, Simon G: New system for non-contact laser photothermal keratoplasty (LPTK). *Proc SPIE* 1877:57–60, 1993.

20. Moreira H, Campos M, Sawusch, McDonnell JM, Sand B, McDonnell PJ: Holmium laser thermokeratoplasty. *Ophthalmol* 100:752–761, 1993.

21. Thompson VM, Seiler T, Durrie DS, Cavanaugh TB: Holmium: YAG laser thermokeratoplasty for hyperopia and astigmatism: an overview. *Refract Corneal Surg* 9:S134–S137, 1993.

22. Durrie DS, Schumer DJ, Cavanaugh TB: Holmium:YAG laser thermokeratoplasty for hyperopia. *J Refract Corneal Surg* 10:S277–S280, 1994.

23. Thompson V: Ho:YAG laser thermokeratoplasty for correction of astigmatism. *J Refract Corneal Surg* 10: S293, 1994.

24. Koch DD, Abarca A, Villarreal R, Menefee RF, Berry MJ, Hennings DR: Six-month follow-up of laser thermal keratoplasty for treatment of hyperopia. *Invest Ophthalmol Vis Sci* 35:1488, 1994.

25. Er H, Menefee RF, Valderrama GL, Anderson JA, Moore M, Koch DD: Acute histopathological changes induced by laser thermal keratoplasty. *Invest Ophthalmol Vis Sci* 35:2021, 1994.

26. Parel JM, Ren Q, Simon G: Noncontact laser photothermal keratoplasty. I: Biophysical principles and laser beam delivery system. *J Refract Corneal Surg* 10: 511–518, 1994.

27. Simon G, Ren Q, Parel JM. Noncontact laser photothermal keratoplasty. II: Refractive effects and treatment parameters in cadaver eyes. *J Refract Corneal Surg* 10:519–528, 1994.

28. Ren Q, Simon G, Parel JM: Noncontact laser photothermal keratoplasty. III: Histological study in animal eyes. *J Refract Corneal Surg* 10:529–539, 1994.

29. Thompson VM: Holmium:YAG laser thermokeratoplasty. Paper presented at American Academy of Ophthalmology meeting, San Francisco, CA, 3 November 1994.

30. Cherry PMH: Holmium:YAG laser to treat astigmatism associated with myopia and hyperopia. *J Refract Surg* 11:S349–S357, 1995.

31. Hennekes R: Holmium:YAG laser thermokeratoplasty for correction of astigmatism. *J Refract Surg* 11:S358–S360, 1995.

32. Ariyasu RG, Sand B, Menefee R, Hennings D, Rose C, Berry M, Garbus JJ, McDonnell PJ: Holmium laser thermal keratoplasty of 10 poorly sighted eyes. *J Refract Surg* 11:358–365, 1995.

33. Koch DD, Villarreal R, Abarca A, Menefee RF, Kohnen T, Vassiliadis A, Berry M: Hyperopia correction by noncontact holmium:YAG laser thermal keratoplasty: clinical study with 2-year follow-up. *Ophthalmol* 103(5):731–45 May 1996.

34. Koch DD, Kohnen T, McDonnell PJ, Menefee RF, Berry MJ: Hyperopia correction by noncontact holmium:YAG laser thermal keratoplasty: U.S. phase IIa clinical study with 1-year follow-up. *Ophthalmol* 103(10):1525–35, Oct 1996.

35. Koch DD, Kohnen T, Anderson JA, et al: Histological changes and wound healing response following 10-pulse noncontact holmium:YAG laser thermal keratoplasty. *J Refract Surg* 12:in press, 1996.

36. Kohnen T, Husain SE, Koch DD: Corneal topography following noncontact Ho:YAG laser thermal keratoplasty. *J Cataract Refract Surg* 22:427–435, 1996.

37. Kohnen T, Koch DD McDonnell PJ, et al: Hyperopia correction by noncontact holmium:YAG laser thermal keratoplasty: U.S. phase IIa clinical study with 18-month follow-up. To be submitted to *Klin Monatsbl Augenheilkd*, 1996.

38. Villarreal RV, Koch DD, Kohnen T, et al: Hyperopia correction by noncontact holmium:YAG laser thermal keratoplasty: 5 pulse treatments with 1-year follow-up. To be submitted to *J Refract Surg*, 1996.

39. Azzolini M, Vinciguerra P, Epstein D, Prussiani A, Radice P: Laser thermokeratoplasty for the correction of hyperopia: a comparison of two different application patterns. *Invest Ophthalmol Vis Sci* 36:S716, 1995.

40. Kohnen T, Koch DD, Anderson JA, et al: Histological changes and wound healing response following 5-pulse noncontact holmium:YAG laser thermal keratoplasty. To be submitted to *Invest Ophthalmol Vis Sci*, 1996.

41. George SP, Johnson DG, Ashton J: Holmium:YAG laser thermokeratoplasty post-PRK. Paper presented at Pacific Coast Symposium on Refractive Surgery, Whistler, British Columbia, Canada, February 1996.

42. Herse P, Siu A: Short-term effects of proparacaine on human corneal thickness. *Acta Ophthalmol* 70:740–744, 1992.

43. Uozato H, Guyton D, Waring GO III. Centering corneal surgical procedures. In Waring GO III, ed: *Refractive Keratotomy for Myopia and Astigmatism*. St. Louis, MO, Mosby-Year Book, 1992, pp491–505.

44. Waxler M, Drum B, Lin S, et al: Refractive Surgery Lasers: Consensus on Clinical Issues. Rockville, MD, Center for Devices and Radiological Health, draft document dated February 28, 1996.

45. Leibowitz M, Krueger DE, Maunder LR, Milton RC, Kini MM, Kahn HA, Nickerson RJ, Pool J, Colton TL, Ganley JP, Lowenstern JJ, Dawber TR: The Framingham Eye Study Monograph. VIII. Visual Acuity. *Surv Ophthalmol* 24(Suppl):472–479, 1980.

46. O'Brart DPS, Lohmann CP, Fitzke FW, Klonos G, Corbett MC, Kerr-Muir MG, Marshall J: Disturbances in night vision after excimer laser photorefractive keratectomy. *Eye* 8:46–51, 1994.

CHAPTER 15

The Use of the Non-Contact Holmium-YAG Laser for the Correction of Primary Hyperopia, Post-PRK Hyperopia, and Post-LASIK Hyperopia: Canadian Experience Using the Sunrise Technologies System

Louis E. Probst
Jeffery J. Machat

INTRODUCTION

Thermal keratoplasty alters the anterior corneal curvature by heating the stromal tissue to 60–65°C[1] causing collagen to shrink to 30–50% of its original length,[2] for up to 90% of the stromal thickness.[3,4] At higher temperatures, substantial additional shrinkage does not occur, however thermal injury and necrosis can result[4] and this may be a factor in the long-term hyperopic regressive effects noted following thermal keratoplasty. This thermal processing of collagen produces dissociation of hydrogen bonds, partial unwinding and coiling of the triple helix, cross-linking between amino acid moieties, and changes in stromal hydration.[5] Whereas the collagen of normal corneas has a half-life of approximately 20 years, the effect of collagen turnover on the long-term stability of thermal keratoplasty is unknown.[5] The Sunrise Holmium:YAG laser system offers the accuracy of laser technology to the application of corneal thermal keratoplasty.

HISTORICAL REVIEW

Thermal keratoplasty has been performed in the past using a variety of techniques including heated object, microwaves, and most recently lasers. Lans[6] was the first to study cautery in rabbit corneas in 1898. Rowsey and Doss[7] attempted thermal kerato-

plasty with a radio frequency probe however this work was abandoned due to poor predictability. Fyodorov[8] devised the technique of inserting a heated needle into the stroma to produce temperatures of 600°C. Unfortunately, this method also suffered from regression and poor predictability and is no longer performed. The Holmium:YAG laser offers the latest method of thermal keratoplasty. Advantages of laser thermal keratoplasty (LTK) include the excellent penetration of the laser wavelength into the cornea, relatively low cost, and the ease of use.[9]

Histopathological studies of the treated cornea after LTK have identified increased epithelial eosinophilia and hyperplasia with elongated nuclei,[4] increased hematoxylin uptake with a loss of distinct stromal lamellae[4] and no stromal necrosis.[2] No morphological effects have been found on the endothelial cell structures of human corneas at the common energy densities used.[2] The maximal endothelial loss caused by LTK on the rabbit cornea, which is only 65% the thickness of the human cornea, was found to be 1.2% with an irradiance pattern of 32 spots at maximal laser fluence levels (≥ 20 J/cm^2).[4]

The basic pattern for the treatment spots of the Holmium:YAG laser involves eight radial sites spread over 360° in an octagonal pattern with the spots 45° apart. Seiler and coworkers have identified a linear relationship between the clear zone diameter and the refractive change with approximately 5.0 D of myopic change at 5.0 mm and only 1.0 D of change at 9.0 mm.[9] Koch and coworkers have found that treatment pattern diameters 3.5 mm or less flatten the cornea centrally whereas diameters 6.0 to 7.0 mm steepen the central cornea and between 3.5 to 5.5 mm there is a "null zone" that produces little persistent change in corneal curvature.[10,11] Multiple rings of treatment can be applied at different diameters for higher degrees of hyperopia.[12] A radial pattern of multiple LTK rings of different diameters has been found to achieve a significantly better refractive outcome and faster visual rehabilitation than a skew pattern.[13] Astigmatic LTK steepens the flat corneal meridian by positioning the four to eight variable diameter treatment spots separated by 45° so that they straddle the flat corneal axis. With astigmatic LTK there is an associated steepening of the central cornea with a resultant hyperopic correction of 0.5 D for every 1.0 D of astigmatism correction.[9]

Currently, LTK is performed clinically with holmium doped yttrium aluminum garnet (Ho:YAG) lasers that are available in the contact (Summit Technology, Inc., Waltham, Mass) and the noncontact (Sunrise Technologies, Inc., Fremont, Calif) varieties. The Summit Ho:YAG system emits the 2.06 μm wavelength with 300 microsecond pulses at a 15 Hz repetition frequency and a pulse energy of approximately 19 mJ. Each treatment location receives 25 pulses. The laser is delivered through a fiber-optic hand piece focused with a sapphire tip that is applied to the corneal surface producing a 700 μm diameter treatment spot to a depth of approximately 450 μm or 80% of the average corneal thickness.[9] The Sunrise Ho:YAG system is a compact solid-state laser which emits the 2.13 μm wavelength with 250 microsecond pulses at a 5 Hz repetition frequency with pulse energies from 8 to 11 J/cm^2.[11] One to eight pulse exposures of 220 to 240 mJ can be applied to each treatment location and this produces a 500 to 600 μm spot[11] that extends to about 420 μm or 75% of the corneal thickness.[2]

Durrie and coworkers[12] have reported follow-up data on eyes treated with the Summit Ho:YAG laser. A total of 79% of eyes with preoperative hyperopia between 2.0 to 6.62 D were within one diopter of the intended correction and 75% achieved J2 or better near vision at 6 months follow-up. Two lines of best corrected visual acuity were

lost by 7% of patients due to irregular astigmatism. Regression patterns stabilized at the 6 month follow-up however regression was identified in some patients at one year.[14] Small studies of the treatment of astigmatism have demonstrated continued regression even one year after treatment that in some cases resulted in keratometry values returning to their pretreatment values.[15,16] Regression was particularly noted in hyperopic astigmatism, younger patients, and larger amounts of myopic astigmatism.[16]

The studies of the Sunrise Ho:YAG LTK have found an initial hyperopic reduction of 1.4 D at three months.[17] Ismail found that 21% of eyes had virtually total regression of refractive correction at 15 months after surgery.[18] Pop and Arus found significant regression in the hyperopic correction up to six months postoperatively leaving an average of 1.2 D of correction with similar regression of astigmatic correction, however 80% of eyes had a correction of at least one diopter at one year.[19] A strong correlation was found between the age of the patient and the degree of correction attained.[19] Koch and coworkers have reported two year posttreatment results after spherical hyperopic LTK with the Sunrise Ho:YAG laser on 21 eyes.[5,20] The four eyes with clear zone diameters less than 6.0 mm had no long term correction. The remaining eyes (n = 17) were treated with a 6.0 mm clear zone diameter, 10 pulses, 8 spots, and pulse radiant energies of 7.5–9.0 J/cm^2. The mean change in the refraction in this group was −0.79 ± 0.74 D with a mean change in astigmatism of 0.1 D at 18 month follow-up[16] and a mean regression of only 0.1 D between three months and 0.2 D at two years postoperatively.[21] Mean uncorrected visual acuity improved from 20/150 to 20/50. No patient lost two or more lines of Snellen visual acuity and the only complication was an increase of refractive astigmatism of 0.5–1.0 D in four patients.

FDA Phase 2A studies with one year follow-up using modified protocols of two treatment rings at 6 and 7 mm with 10 pulses achieved a mean correction of 1.7 D.[5] Further modification of the treatment variables using three rings with only five pulse treatments gave 3.5 D of correction at six months follow-up.[5] Koch and coworkers have recently reported data for a group of 12 patients with an average age of 57 years that suggested that two radial rings of five pulses placed at 5.0 and 6.0 mm using 240 mJ provides the ideal refractive effect of noncontact Ho:YAG,[22] however further study in a larger and younger group of patients will be required to fully evaluate this technique.

There has been a paucity of information presented or published on the efficacy of Ho:YAG LTK for the treatment of the iatrogenic hyperopia that occasionally occurs following PRK and LASIK. Sunrise Ho:YAG LTK has been found to produce an average change of 3.6 D at 12 months with 21–63% regression from the initial postoperative correction when used to treat post-PRK hyperopia.[23] Johnson and coworkers have presented 43 post-PRK hyperopic eyes that obtained an average myopic shift of 2.72 D at 6 months with 0.49 D of regression.[24] The absence of Bowman's membrane and the thinner central cornea following PRK have been proposed as conditions which may increase the efficacy and stability of Ho:YAG LTK.[23]

CURRENT SURGICAL TECHNIQUE

The two authors (LEP and JJM) performed all the procedures with the Sunrise Ho:YAG gLase 210 laser system using the technique that has been previously described.[25] Generally, unilateral procedures were performed however bilateral treatment is definitely possible because of the quick and painless nature of the procedure and the rapid 24 to 48 hour recovery of the corneal epithelium. Initially patients are fully informed of the risks of the procedure and sign a detailed consent form. We provided a detailed description of the procedure itself including the beeping noise the Sunrise system makes when it is in the "ready" mode to alleviate any patient anxiety during the procedure. The eye(s) were thoroughly anesthetized with multiple applications of 0.5% proparacaine and one drop of Tobradex starting 15 minutes prior to the procedure. The laser system was calibrated and the centration of the eight red helium-neon (wavelength 632 nm) aiming beams were checked prior to each treatment session.

The entire procedure usually took only a few minutes to perform. A wire nonadjustable speculum was inserted and the patient was seated at the Nikon slit-lamp biomicroscope delivery system. The eye was left open for two to three minutes for the tear film to dry or alternatively in some cases, compressed air was used to uniformly dry the cornea tear film. The endpoint of corneal dryness is reached when a mottled reflection is visible with cobalt blue filter illumination. A dry cornea is essential to allow the appropriate thermal effect to be derived from the Ho:YAG laser application.

The spot center diameters were adjusted to 6.75–7.25 mm for a single ring, 6.50–6.75 and 7.0–7.5 mm for two rings, and 6.25, 6.75–7.0, and 7.25–7.5 mm for three rings. Astigmatism was treated by blocking four of the eight spots and treating with remaining four spots straddling the minus axis and a spot diameter of 6.25–7.0 mm. One ring of spots was applied for each 1.25–1.5 diopters of hyperopia and four minus axis straddling spots were applied for each diopter of astigmatism. Multiple treatment rings were applied initially in a staggered fashion and later in a radial fashion. Seven to eight pulses were applied with pulse energies set between 220 and 240 mJ.

The patient was asked to fixate on the red fixation light and gentle but firm head support was applied by an assistant in order to minimize head movement during the brief period of laser energy application. The intersecting green helium neon (wavelength 543) beams were brought together and centered on the pupil. The "aiming" mode provided the visualization of the eight red helium neon placement beams that indicated the placement positions of the Ho:YAG laser spots and allowed further verification of the accuracy of centration (Fig. 15–1). The entire duration of actual laser treatment was less than two seconds for each eye.

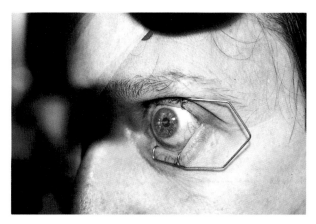

Fig. 15–1. With a speculum placed in the eye, the green helium neon aiming beams are focused on the cornea and the peripheral helium neon placement beams are checked for centration prior to the application of Sunrise Ho:YAG LTK.

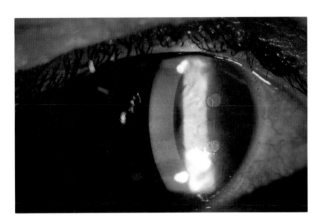

Fig. 15–2. Appearance of the cornea, one day postoperatively after a double ring of Sunrise Ho:YAG LTK has been applied to the cornea at 6.75 and 7.50 mm. The white spots represent the areas of the thermal effects of the laser. Between the spots, a ring of anterior stromal striae can be observed indicating that the Sunrise Ho:YAG LTK treatment was effective.

Following the procedure the speculum was removed and the treated eye received an additional drop of proparacaine and a drop of Tobradex. The patient was then instructed to use Tobradex four times a day for the next week. The patients were followed 24 hours, one week, and then monthly after surgery. The white spots from the Sunrise Ho:YAG LTK slowly fade over the next few postoperative months (Figs. 15–2 and 15–3).

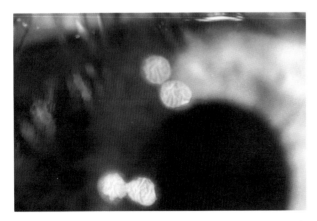

Fig. 15–3. One day postoperative appearance of a double ring of Sunrise Ho:YAG LTK with ring diameters of 6.25 and 7.5 mm placed in a radial fashion. The white spots will fade over the next several months.

CLINICAL RESULTS

The results of noncontact Sunrise Ho:YAG LTK for the correction of primary hyperopia, post-PRK hyperopia, and post-LASIK hyperopia at TLC The Laser Center, Windsor, Canada were retrospectively reviewed. A total of 42 eyes of 26 patients with primary hyperopia, 19 eyes of 18 patients with post-PRK hyperopia, and 7 eyes of 7 patients with post-LASIK hyperopia were treated. The eyes were divided into either group A with <2.0 D spherical equivalent subjective manifest refraction (SE SMR) and <1.0 D astigmatism, or group B with between 2.00 and 3.00 D SE SMR and <1.0 D astigmatism, or group C with >3.00 D SE SMR and ≥1.0 astigmatism. Statistical analysis was performed by ANOVA and the Student's t-test and a $p < 0.05$ was considered significant.

In the primary hyperopia group the average preoperative SE SMR was 2.12 D (range: 1.25–4.75 D) and the average age was 50.1 years (range: 29–58 years). The average follow-up was 7.1 months (range: 1–16 months). Ninety-one percent of eyes (21/23) achieved at least 20/40 visual acuity, 78% of eyes (18/23) were within one diopter of emmetropia, and 9% of eyes (2/23) required retreatment in group A. In Group B, 100% of eyes (5/5) achieved at least 20/40 visual acuity, 60% of eyes (3/5) were within one diopter of emmetropia, and 20% of eyes (1/5) required retreatment. In group C, 60% of eyes (9/15) achieved at 20/40 visual acuity, 27% of eyes (4/15) were within one diopter of emmetropia, and 30% of eyes (5/15) required retreatment (Fig. 15–4). The data demonstrate the decrease in the efficacy of the Sunrise Ho:YAG LTK system for the eyes with higher levels of hyperopia and astigmatism (group C) and the greater need for enhancements in this group.

The effect on a single ring of Ho:YAG LTK was evaluated according to the patient age on eyes with less than 1.50 D SE SMR and <1.0 D of astigmatism at 3 months of follow-up (n = 12 patients). The average hyperopic correction in the 45–50 year age group was 1.12 D, in the 51–55 year age group was 1.18 D, and the >55 year age group was 1.75 D. Although the small numbers did not allow a demonstration of statistical significance, the trend in the data is clearly evident with a greater effect of Sunrise Ho:YAG LTK in the older age groups (Fig. 15–5.)

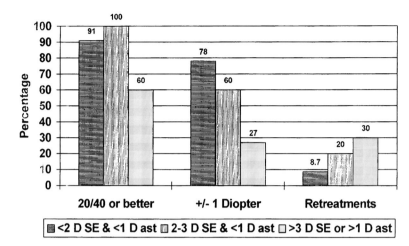

Fig. 15–4. Results of noncontact Ho:YAG LTK for the treatment of 42 eyes with primary hyperopia. The visual results diminish and retreatment rate increased substantially in group C with the greater hyperopia and astigmatism.

All the Sunrise Ho:YAG LTK treatments in the post-PRK patients were performed at least 6 months following the original procedure. The average preoperative SE SMR was 1.99 D (range: 0.38–4.38 D) and the average age was 44.7 years (range: 25–58 years). In group A, the results with follow-up for 3.5 months (range: 1–9 months) indicated that 90% of eyes (9/10) achieved at least 20/40 visual acuity, 80% of eyes (8/10) were within one diopter of emmetropia, and none of the eyes

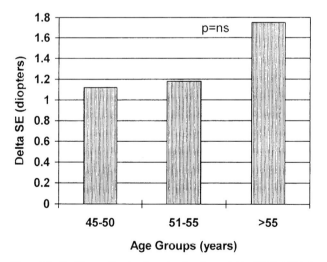

Fig. 15–5. The effect of a single ring of Ho:YAG LTK for some of the eyes of group A (n = 12) is organized according to age group. While not statistically significant, there is a clear trend of an increased effect of Ho:YAG LTK in the >55 year age group.

required retreatment. In group B, 100% of eyes (5/5) achieved at least 20/40 visual acuity, 80% of eyes (4/5) were within one diopter of emmetropia, and 20% of eyes (1/5) required retreatment. In group C, 100% of eyes (4/4) achieved at least 20/40 visual acuity, 25% of eyes (1/4) were within one diopter of emmetropia, and 25% of eyes (1/4) required retreatment (Fig. 15–6). The data illustrate that the visual results of the Sunrise Ho:YAG LTK are impressive for all ranges of post-PRK hyperopia including those eyes in group C with higher degrees of hyperopia and astigmatism, however this group had a greater need of enhancements.

The Sunrise Ho:YAG LTK was performed at least 9 months following the original LASIK procedure to ensure stability of the corneal flap and the refractive status. The average preoperative SE SMR was 1.56 D (range: 0.75–2.5 D) and the average age was 51 years (range: 45–55). Average follow-up was 2.9 months (range: 1–9 months). All eyes in the three groups (7/7) achieved at least 20/40 vision and all except one eye from the three groups (6/7) were within one diopter of emmetropia. No cases required retreatment (Fig. 15–7). This data illustrates that the visual and refractive results of the Sunrise Ho:YAG LTK for the post-LASIK hyperopes are much more impressive than in the primary hyperopia and the post-PRK hyperopia groups, particularly for corrections of higher hyperopia and astigmatism (group C).

In the post-LASIK group, a statistically greater treatment effect was observed that was between 2–3 diopters of hyperopic correction. Unfortunately,

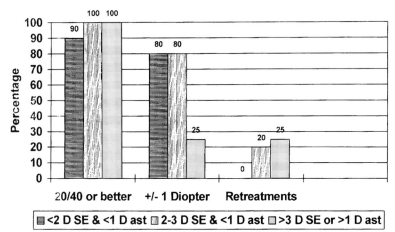

Fig. 15–6. Results of noncontact Ho:YAG LTK for the treatment of 19 eyes with post-PRK hyperopia. The visual results were excellent for all degrees of hyperopia and astigmatism however the retreatment rate increased substantially in group C with the greater hyperopia and astigmatism.

the small numbers and irregular follow-up of this group did not provide sufficient data for a detailed analysis however the trend of the greater effect in these eyes is clearly demonstrated (Figs. 15–8 and 15–9). The increased efficacy of Ho:YAG LTK in the post-PRK eyes was felt to be due to the absence of Bowman's membrane of these corneas.[21] Our data suggest however, that the thickness of the cornea may also be an important variable in the net hyperopic correction after LTK since the post-LASIK corneas had had an average of 121 microns of tissue ablated during the original LASIK procedure. In fact, Mihai Pop, MD has performed phototherapeutic keratectomy to eliminate Bowman's membrane prior to performing Sunrise Ho:YAG

LTK and this did not provide any increase in the effectiveness of the procedure.

Our results indicate that Sunrise noncontact Ho:YAG LTK is particularly effective in correcting primary hyperopia and post-PRK hyperopia with <2.0 D SE SMR and ≤1.0 D astigmatism but far less successful with higher degrees of hyperopia and astigmatism in these groups. Post-LASIK eyes however, appear at achieve good results of the Sunrise Ho:YAG LTK even with the higher degrees of hyperopia and astigmatism.

Our three year experience with the Sunrise Ho:YAG LTK laser has indicated that there are several key factors governing the success of this treatment. Hyperopia less than 2.50 D, patient age

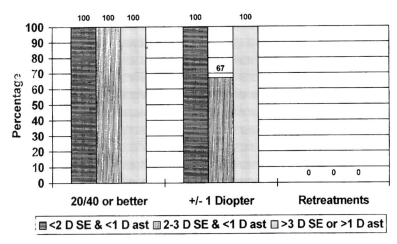

Fig. 15–7. Results of noncontact Ho:YAG LTK for the treatment of 7 eyes with post-LASIK hyperopia. The visual results were excellent for all degrees of hyperopia and astigmatism and no retreatments have been required.

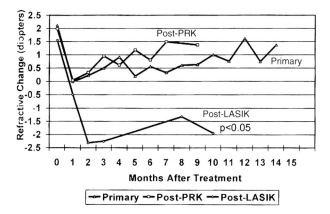

Fig. 15–8. Refractive change from preoperative hyperopia to the postoperative SE SMR values for the primary hyperopia, post-PRK hyperopia, and the post-LASIK hyperopia groups. The increased effectiveness of Sunrise Ho:YAG LTK in the post-LASIK group is well illustrated.

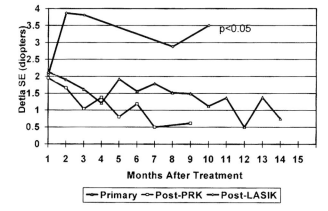

Fig. 15–9. Regression of the postoperative hyperopic correction for the primary hyperopia, post-PRK, and post-LASIK hyperopes. The primary hyperopia and the post-PRK hyperopes experienced over one diopter of regression over the follow-up period. The post-LASIK hyperopes obtained a significantly greater initial hyperopic correction from the Ho:YAG LTK. Further follow-up data will be required to detect regression in the post-LASIK eyes.

greater than 45 years, corneal thickness less than 550 μm, a normal range of corneal curvature (42–45.0 D), and a corneal diameter of at least 11 mm are all ocular characteristics that indicate a favorable outcome. Patients without one or more of these characteristics tend to have less impressive results. Stated another way, hyperopic eyes with extremes of any of the ocular parameters tend to be poor candidates for Sunrise Ho:YAG LTK.

COMPLICATIONS

All patients experience a small degree of foreign body sensation and photophobia for the first 24 to 48 hours following the procedure. No patient experienced a decentration of the treatment ring sufficient to induce irregular astigmatism or alter the refractive result. Patients often initially experienced a monovision phenomena in the treated eye because of the initial overcorrection however all patients were counseled preoperatively that this effect was expected and transient.

Data analysis of the average monthly postoperative SE SMR from the preoperative values indicated regression of the effect of the Ho:YAG LTK in the primary hyperopia and the post-PRK groups (Figs. 15–8 and 15–9). In these groups, the average initial myopic shift was found to be approximately 2 D which regressed to less than one diopter at the last follow-up (Fig. 15–9). In the post-LASIK group, more follow-up data will be required before a regressive effect can be effectively evaluated.

The significant hyperopic regression and undercorrections in primary high hyperopia and the post-PRK high hyperopia groups required retreatments in 9–30% of cases. An increase in astigmatism of greater than one diopter was noted in 9% of all cases and two-thirds of these cases involved hyperopes in group C who required retreatments or greater than two rings of Ho:YAG LTK.

None of the eyes experienced a loss of best corrected visual acuity. None of the post-PRK eyes experienced increased or recurrence of corneal haze. No flap related problems occurred in any of the post-LASIK eyes despite the fact that the single 7.0 mm center diameter Ho:YAG treatment ring that was used in the treatment of all of the post-

LASIK eyes was being placed directly onto the corneal flap which averaged 8.5 mm in diameter.

FUTURE CONSIDERATIONS AND DEVELOPMENTS

Most investigators agree that Ho:YAG LTK is effective for less than 2–3 diopters of primary hyperopia with minimal astigmatism and treatment should be limited to patients 40 years or older.[3,19,26] Since approximately 80% of the hyperopic population has 3.00 D or less, noncontact Ho:YAG could potentially treat most patients in this refractive range.[27] Although persistent regression has been noted, the treatment is relatively easy to perform, post-treatment recovery is fast, and the patient acceptance is high.[3] No vision threatening complications have been reported to date.[5] Further modifications of the treatment parameters that minimize keratocyte injury and maximize collagen shrinkage should improve the long-term regression, efficacy, and predictability of this procedure.[5]

Ho:YAG LTK currently offers the only effective treatment of the iatrogenic hyperopia that occasionally occurs following PRK and LASIK. Patients are extremely grateful when their uncorrected vision improves and appreciate the rapid visual rehabilitation. The multi-focal effect of Ho:YAG LTK provides an additional benefit by increasing the range of useful vision. Further investigation into the effect of corneal thickness on the results of noncontact Ho:YAG LTK will allow greater predictability of the results in post-PRK and post-LASIK cornea. Most surgeons do not recommend Ho:YAG LTK for post-radial keratotomy (RK) hyperopia because of the risk of opening the RK incisions when the stromal tissue contracts.

Scanning spot excimer laser systems with eye tracking technology and new treatment algorithms will permit hyperopic PRK and LASIK to become future methods of choice for the treatment of low to moderate hyperopia but these techniques are currently in their infancy of development when compared to the progress that has been made in the treatment of myopia.

REFERENCES

1. Shaw EL, Gasset AR: Thermokeratoplasty (TKP) temperature profile. *Invest Ophthalmol* 13;181–186, 1974.

2. Ariyasu RG, Sand B, Menefee R, Hennings D, Rose C, Berry M, Garbus, JJ, McDonnell PJ: Holmium laser thermal keratoplasty of 10 poorly sighted eyes. *J Refract Surg* 11:358–365, 1995.

3. Yanoff M: Holmium laser hyperopia thermokeratoplasty update. *Eur J Implant Ref Surg* 7:89–91, 1995.

4. Moreira H, Campos M, Sawusch MR, McDonnell JM, Sand B, McDonnell PJ: Holmium laser thermokeratoplasty. *Ophthalmology* 100:752–761, 1993.

5. Koch DD: Holmium laser thermal keratoplasty with slit-lamp delivery system. *Am Acad Ophthalmol Meeting*, Atlanta, Georgia, October 30–November 3, 1995.

6. Lans LJ: Experimentelle Untersuchungen uber die Entstehung von Astigmatismus durch nicht-perforierende Corneawunden. *Graefes Arch Clin Ophthalmol* 45:117–152, 1898.

7. Rowsey JJ: Electrosurgical keratoplasty: update and retraction. *Invest Ophthalmol Vis Sci* 28:224, 1987.

8. Fyodorov SN: A new technique for the treatment of hyperopia. In Schachar RA, Levy NS, Schachar L (eds): *Keratorefractive Surgery*, Denison, Texas, LAL Publishing, 1989.

9. Thompson VM, Seiler T, Durrie DS, Cavanaugh TB: Holmium:YAG laser thermokeratoplasty for hyperopia and astigmatism: an overview. *Refract Corneal Surg* 9(Suppl.):S134–S137, 1993.

10. Koch DD, Abarca A, Menefee RF: Ho:YAG laser thermal keratoplasty (LTK) for corrections of spherical refractive errors. Current Research: *Refractive and Cataract Surgery Symposium*. Minneapolis, Minnesota, November, 1993.

11. Koch DD, Berry MJ, Vassiliadis A, Abarca AA, Villarreal R, Haft ED: Noncontact Holmium:YAG laser thermal keratoplasty. In Salz JJ (ed): *Corneal Laser Surgery*, St. Louis, Mosby, 1995.

12. Durrie DS, Schumer J, Cavanaugh TB: Holmium: YAG laser thermokeratoplasty for hyperopia. *J Refract Corneal Surg* 10(Suppl.):S227–S280, 1994.

13. Azzolini M, Vinciguerra P, Epstein D, Prussiani A, Radice P: Laser thermokeratoplasty for the correction of hyperopia. A comparison of two differ-

ent application patterns. *Invest Ophthalmol Vis Sci* 36(4):S716, 1995.

14. Yanoff M. Holmium laser hyperopia thermokeratoplasty update. *Eur J Implant Ref Surg* 7:89–91, 1995.

15. Hennekes R. Holmium:YAG laser thermokeratoplasty for correction of astigmatism. *J Refract Surg* 11(Suppl.):S358–S360, 1995.

16. Cherry PMH: Holmium:YAG laser to treat astigmatism associated with myopia or hyperopia. *J Refract Surg* 11(Suppl.):S349–S357, 1995.

17. Fucigna RJ, Gelber E, Belmont S: Laser thermal keratoplasty for the correction of hyperopia: a retrospective study of 35 patients. *1995 ISRS Pre-Academy Conference and Exhibition*, Atlanta, Georgia, October 26, 1995.

18. Ismail MM: Non-contact LTK by holmium laser for hyperopia: 15 months follow-up. *1995 ISRS Mid-Summer Symposium and Exhibition*, Minneapolis, Minnesota, July 28–30, 1995.

19. Pop M, Aras M: Regression after hyperopic correction with the holmium laser: one year follow-up. *1995 Mid-Summer Symposium and Exhibition*, Minneapolis, Minnesota, July 28–30, 1995.

20. Koch DD, Villarreal R, Abarca A, Menefee RF, Berry MJ: Two-year follow-up of holmium:YAG thermal keratoplasty for the treatment of hyperopia. *Invest Ophthalmol Vis Sci* 36(4):S2, 1995.

21. Koch DD, Abarca A, Villarreal R, Menefee R, Kohnen T, Vassiliadis A, Berry M: Hyperopia correction by noncontact holmium:YAG laser thermal keratoplasty. Clinical results with two year follow-up. *Ophthalmology*:103:731–740, 1996.

22. Koch DD, Villarreal R, Kohnen T, McDonnell PJ, Vinciguerra P, Menefee R, Berry M: Intrastromal procedures: The use of the noncontact holmium: YAG laser for correction of hyperopia—Sunrise Technologies experience. In Sher NA (ed): *Refractive Surgery of Hyperopia and Presbyopia*. Baltimore, Williams & Wilkins 1997.

23. Alio JL, Ismail M: Management of post-PRK hyperopia by holmium laser. *1995 ISRS Pre-Academy Conference and Exhibition*, Atlanta, Georgia, October 26, 1995.

24. George SP, Johnson DG, Ashton J: Hyperopia correction by noncontact Ho:YAG thermal keratoplasty of eyes with overcorrected photorefractive keratectomy for myopia compared to naturally occurring hyperopia. *ASCRS Symposium on Cataract, IOL, and Refractive Surgery*. Seattle, Washington, June 1996.

25. Maschat JJ: Postoperative PRK Management. In Machat JJ (ed): *Excimer Laser Refractive Surgery*. Thorofare, NJ, Slack, 1996.

26. Mathys B, Van Horenbeeck R: Contact holmium laser thermokeratoplasty (LTK) for hyperopia surgery: follow-up of our first clinical cases. *1995 ISRS Pre-Academy Conference and Exhibition*, Atlanta, Georgia, October 26, 1995.

27. Leibowitz M, Krueger DE, Maunder LR, Maunder LR, Milton RC, Kini MM, Kahn HA, Nickerson RJ, Pool J, Colton TL, Ganley JP, Lowenstein JJ, Dawber TR: The Framingham Eye Study Monograph VIII. Visual acuity. *Surv Ophthalmol* 24(Suppl):472–470, 1980.

section V

Intrastromal Procedures

B. Contact

CHAPTER 16

Holmium: Yag Laser Thermokeratoplasty: The Summit System

Vance Thompson

INTRODUCTION

Prior to the development of the holmium:YAG laser to perform collagen shrinkage, the most popular technique utilized to steepen corneal curvature was radial thermokeratoplasty (RTK). RTK was developed and popularized by Fyodorov.[1] An inherent lack of predictability and a high incidence of regression accompanied the RTK procedure and limited its growth as a refractive option to lessen hyperopia.[2] Interestingly enough, the first attempts to heat collagen were performed in the late 1800s with the Dutch ophthalmologist Lans being the first to publish experiments utilizing heat on the cornea to induce changes in corneal curvature.[3]

It has been theorized that utilizing the holmium:YAG laser to heat the cornea represented an advancement in corneal collagen shrinkage with hopes of increased predictability and a lessened incidence of regression when compared to the RTK technique.[4] This goal has been partially realized, although some of the limitations seen with other forms of collagen shrinkage have shown themselves over time to be limitations in the holmium technique also, namely, regression of refractive effect over time.[5]

THE PHYSIOLOGY OF COLLAGEN SHRINKAGE

Corneal collagen fibrils shrink rapidly (to about one-third of their original length) due to unraveling of the helical structure when exposed to heat.[6] The exact temperature at which the cornea needs to be heated for this shrinking phenomena to occur is around 55–60°C. Once collagen is heated to levels higher than the 75° range, heat labile crosslinks in the collagen complex are damaged and collagen

relaxation occurs. Lower temperatures than this (55° to 60° range) show minimal collagen shrinkage changes. Higher temperatures will, again, cause relaxation of the collagen fibrils with even higher temperatures causing necrosis of the collagen. The point being that when performing collagen shrinkage procedures you want to elevate the corneal temperature enough to cause collagen shrinkage, but not high enough to cause relaxation or necrosis of the collagen and thus lessen the potential effect.

It appears that one of the problems encountered in the Fyodorov RTK technique was the use of a nicrome wire probe positioned at 90% corneal depth and heated to 600°C. These extreme temperatures lead to heating of the surrounding collagen to temperatures significantly higher than that recommended for collagen shrinkage—the result being relaxation of collagen heated to greater than 70° and necrosis of collagen immediately adjacent to the 600° probe. These high temperatures worked against the collagen shrinkage that was also occurring and contributed to unpredictable results and a high incidence of regression of effect.

THE HOLMIUM:YAG LASER

The holmium:YAG laser is a solid state laser that emits radiation in the infrared region of the electromagnetic spectrum (2.06 microns). This wavelength of laser energy is ideal for heating the corneal water, which in turn heats up the surrounding collagen fibrils and results in a shrinkage effect. The Summit Technology, Inc. holmium:YAG laser (see Fig. 16–1) operates in a pulsed mode. Each pulse has a duration of 300 microseconds. The repetition rate is 15 hertz and the energy delivered per pulse is 19 mJ. We have utilized an energy delivery that

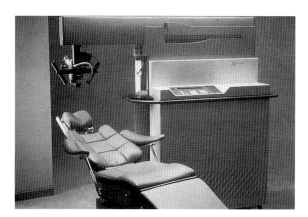

Fig. 16–1 The Summit Technology, Inc. combined excimer/holmium:YAG laser refractive workstation.

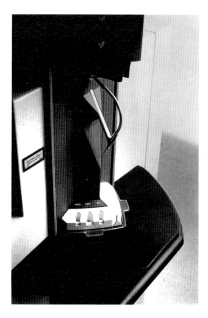

Fig. 16–2 The quartz fiberoptic cable and hand-piece

provides for 25 pulses at each treatment location. The total number of pulses at each treatment location raise the stromal temperature at that spot approximately 50–60°C. This is not a linear relationship (i.e., temperature increase per pulse) but rather additive with the ending pulses at a treatment location providing more of a temperature increase than the beginning pulses. It averages out to be about 2°C temperature elevation per pulse.

There are several characteristics that make this laser ideal for collagen shrinkage. The parameters of pulse duration, repetition rate, energy per pulse, and the number of pulses delivered at a given treatment site are all adjustable. Thus, the ideal temperature elevation can be titrated to a level that optimizes collagen shrinkage without heating too much and without causing relaxation of the collagen, or worse, necrosis of stromal tissue.[7]

The other attraction of this wavelength is that it can be delivered along a quartz fiberoptic if so desired, which is the delivery system that the Summit holmium laser utilizes (*see* Fig. 16–2). In this system, a sapphire focusing tip (Fig. 16–3), with a cone angle 120°, is used to focus the energy a safe distance anterior to Descemet's membrane (*see* Fig. 16–4). This sapphire tip is placed directly on the corneal surface. That is why this form of thermokeratoplasty is termed the contact method (*see* Fig. 16–5), versus the noncontact method developed around a slit-lamp delivery system.[8] The typical cone is approximately 450 microns in depth with a diameter of 700 microns at the corneal surface. This wedge shaped contraction of collagen functions

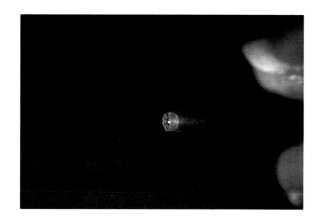

Fig. 16–3 Specially designed sapphire tip which focuses the holmium energy with its cone shaped characteristics.

Fig. 16–4 Wedge shaped zone of collagen shrinkage focused well before Descemet's membrane.

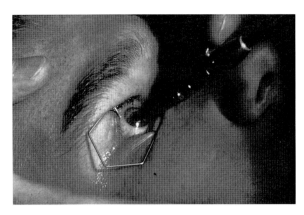

Fig. 16–5 Sapphire focusing tip is placed directly in contact with the patient's cornea at the desired treatment location.

much like a wedge resection of the cornea resulting in a flattening effect at the treatment site (in general the mid-peripheral cornea) with a relative steepening effect away from the treatment site (i.e., the central cornea).

CURRENT TECHNIQUE

Laser Thermokeratoplasty for Hyperopia and Astigmatism

The main refractive indication for performing collagen shrinkage with the holmium laser (technically known as laser thermokeratoplasty or LTK) is to lessen hyperopia. In the LTK procedure, special markers (*see* Fig. 16–6) are used to place equally

spaced marks at variable optical zones (*see* Fig. 16–7).

The optical zone is an important parameter to understand in LTK. One just needs to keep in mind that at (and directly around) the treatment site, the holmium spot causes a flattening effect. You have to get a few millimeters away from the treatment site before a relative steepening effect is noticed. In general, optical zones of 6.0 mm or larger are needed to achieve a central steepening. Optical zones around the 5.0 mm zone give somewhat of a variable response, but in general this zone is considered a "null" zone with theoretically minimal refractive effect obtained. Zones smaller than 5.0 mm begin to not only flatten at the treatment site, but also flatten the central cornea that would make hyperopia worse or myopia better. Some have advocated the holmium as a viable treatment option for the treatment of myopia. This author believes that the risks of putting collagen shrinkage spots at a 4.0 mm optical zone (which is only 2.0 mm from the center of the corena) should be considered. Thus the holmium laser should mainly be limited to the treatment of hyperopia or astigmatism.

Astigmatism treatments with the holmium laser consist of placing the collagen shrinkage zones in the mid-peripheral cornea in the flat axis of astigmatism (the opposite of astigmatic keratotomy-AK). The LTK spots will steepen the flat axis astigmatism. The LTK spots not only steepen the flat axis, they induce a steepening of the overall cornea thus lessening hyperopia (or increasing myopia). The astigmatic LTK procedure is an option for those patients with hyperopic astigmatism. The hyperopic

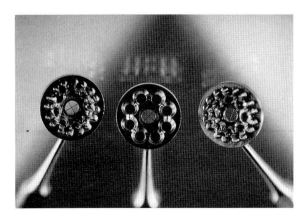

Fig. 16–6 Example of markers designed for performance of LTK.

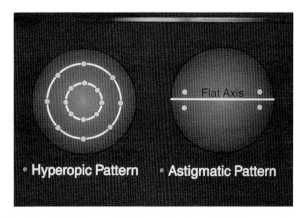

Fig. 16–7 Pattern of LTK spots placed for hyperopia or astigmatism.

reduction in spherical equivalent is typically about 30–40% of the reduction in the astigmatic component of the refraction. Studies have been encouraging for this group of patients.[5] It is a particularly nice option for the hyperopic astigmat due to the fact that performing a pure astigmatic keratotomy in this group would either not change or increase the hyperopic portion of the refractive error.

LTK Technique

Preoperatively the patient receives topical anesthetic and antibiotic starting one half hour before the procedure. They are positioned under the laser and a lid speculum is placed. The procedure is centered on the center of the entrance pupil. The corneal mark is placed in the hyperopia procedure with a marker that leaves an imprint of eight, or sixteen, semicircles at a designated optical zone (or optical zones in the case of sixteen marks). Marker dye can be helpful for visualizing the marks. The contact probe is then positioned in one of the semicircles making sure to keep the probe perpendicular with the corneal surface. It is important for the surgeon to apply slight pressure to nullify any of the surgeon's physiologic tremor. At this point the foot pedal is depressed and the laser energy delivered. It takes slightly under two seconds for the energy delivery. The contraction lines of collagen shrinkage can actually be visualized during the energy delivery. This process is repeated at the remaining seven marked semicircles. After completion of the procedure, the epithelium over the treatment location is noted to be coagulated and is brushed off with a microsponge. This facilitates re-epithelialization which typically takes about two to three days.

During the first few days after the procedure, antibiotic ointment is used until the epithelium is intact. These patients do not typically experience much pain so routine pain control is not needed. Occasionally an oral pain reliever is needed. The treatment spots appear quite opaque with a gradual lessening of the opaqueness over the next two years (*see* Fig. 16–8). Since the refractive effect will regress fairly impressively over the first year, a myopic shift is noted early on. Since it is typically presbyopes undergoing the procedure, they actually find benefit in this newfound reading ability with a gradual improvement in their distance vision.

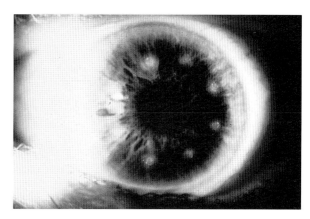

Fig. 16–8 Hyperopic LTK six months postop.

RESULTS OF CLINICAL TRIALS

For refractive purposes, the holmium:YAG laser is still considered investigational in the United States. Summit Technology's United States holmium LTK clinical trials are currently in phase III. Phases I and II have been completed. A number of things have been learned over our four years experience with the LTK procedure. First, young collagen has a tendency to "spring" back to its original shape as evidenced by a rapid regression of effect over the first postoperative year. It is felt that this is a procedure for mature collagen and, as a result, is best reserved for patients above 40 years of age. In general, the older the patient, the more initial effect achieved and the less the long-term regression. Four years ago we predicted, based on European studies, that this would be a procedure for patients with 5 diopters or less of hyperopia.[4] Based on our long-term experience, we have essentially dropped a diopter from our initial predictions as we witnessed fairly impressive regression. Currently the LTK procedure appears to be a reasonable option in patients who are in the presbyopic age group with no more than 2.0 diopters of hyperopia and preferably less than 1.0 diopters. With a quite maximal LTK procedure, the patients in this group should end up with about a 1.0 diopter of residual steepening after two years. The two year results of 17 patients in our phase II clinical trials are shown in Fig. 16–9. The predictability of the LTK procedure in these 17 patients with two-year follow-up is as follows: +0.50 to −0.50 diopters = 23.5%, −0.51 to −1.0

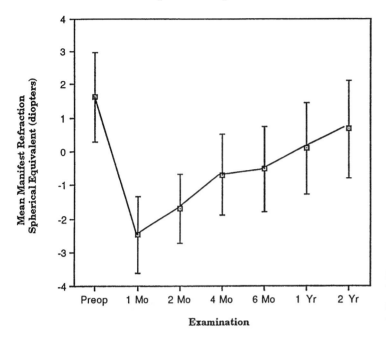

Holmium Hyperopia
Mean Spherical Equivalent vs. Time

Fig. 16–9 Two years results of Summit Technology's United States holmium:YAG Phase II clinical trials. On average, a residual effect of a little over 1.0 diopters of effect is noted.

diopters = 5.9%, −1.1 to −2.0 diopters = 29.4%, and −2.1 to −3.0 diopters = 41.2%. Best corrected vision changes in the 17 patients with two years of follow-up included 14 eyes (82.3%) with no change, 1 eye (5.9%) with an increase in two lines, 1 eye (5.9%) had a decrease in two lines (from 20/12.5 to 20/20), and 1 eye (5.9%) with a decrease of three lines of best corrected visual acuity (20/12.5 to 20/25).

Complications included an induction of astigmatism in many patients. Induced astigmatism (>1.0 D) was reported in five patients (20.8%) at six months, one patient (5.3%) at one year, and one patient (5.9%) at the two-year postoperative visit. It is noteworthy that much of the induced astigmatism still present at six months postoperatively was gone at the one-year visit. We feel it is important to not treat any induced cylinder unless it is persistent and unchanging at the one-year visit. As far as other complications, there was no significant endothelial cell loss, bacterial keratitis, corneal decompensation, or long-term foreign body sensation. Glare was reported in two patients (8.3%) at six months and in no patients at the one-year or longer postoperative visits.

CONCLUSION

The holmium:YAG laser is an effective tool for steepening the cornea. It appears to be an advancement in the field of collagen shrinkage procedures. It is a procedure that should be considered investigational with the main parameters in patient selection being patient age (>40 years) and level of preoperative hyperopia (less than 2.0 diopters). For LTK to survive in the long run and become a mainstream refractive option, advancements are needed in the areas of predictability and stability (probably impossible). This procedure appears to have an acceptable safety profile. But the fact remains that other procedures, such as excimer hyperopic ablations, are making large advancements in the area of hyperopic corrections with promise of greater predictability and stability. In light of the long-term studies on the LTK procedures, and with recent advancements in other areas of hyperopic correction, it appears that the use of the holmium:YAG laser in refractive surgery will most likely not reach the potential that was once hoped unless a more predictable and stable treatment effect is ultimately obtained.

REFERENCES

1. Neumann AC, Fyodorov S, Sanders DR: Radial thermokeratoplasty for the correction of hyperopia. *Refract Corneal Surg* 6:404–412, 1990.
2. Feldman ST, Ellis W, Frucht-Perry J, et al: Regression of effect following radial thermokeratoplasty in humans. *Refract Corneal Surg* 5:288–291, 1989.
3. Lans LJ: Experimentelle untersuchungen uber entstehung von astigmatisumus durch nicht-perforirende Corneawunden Graefes. *Arch Ophthalmol* 44:117–152, 1889.
4. Seiler T, Matallana M, Bende T: Laser thermokeratoplasty by means if a pulsed holmium:YAG laser for hyperopic correction. *Refract Corneal Surg* 6:335–339, 1990.
5. Thompson VM, Seiler T, Duries DS, et al: Holmium:YAG laser thermokeratoplasty for hyperopia and astigmatism. An overview. Supplement to *Refract Corneal Surg* 9:S134–S137, 1993.
6. Allain JC, Lous LE, Cohen-Solal: Isometric tensions developed during the hydrothermal swelling of rat skin. *Connective Tissue Res* 7:127–133, 1980.
7. Thompson VM: Holmium:YAG laser thermokeratoplasty utilizing the Summit System. In Salz JJ, McDonnell PJ, McDonald MB, ed: *Corneal Laser Surgery*, St. Louis, MO, Mosby-Year Book, 1995.
8. Koch DD, Berry MJ, Vassiliadis A, et al: Noncontact holmium-YAG laser thermal keratoplasty. In Salz JJ, McDonnell PJ, McDonald MB, ed: *Corneal Laser Surgery*, St. Louis, MO, Mosby-Year Book, 1995.

CHAPTER 17

Conductive Keratoplasty for the Correction of Hyperopia

Dr. Antonio Mendez G.
Dr. Antonio Mendez Noble

INTRODUCTION

Nonincisionial approaches to refractive surgery have been developed such as the Holmium laser, the excimer laser and now LASIK. These approaches have been explored in the quest of finding a satisfactory solution to hyperopia.

Since April 1993, we have been working with a different approach—a variation of thermokeratoplasty we call Conductive Keratoplasty (CK). This procedure involves working with high frequency current to contract collagen fibers in the cornea and produce steepening of the central area. CK has also evolved through the years.

HISTORICAL REVIEW OF CURRENT TECHNIQUE

Since the nineteenth century, with the pioneering experiments of Lans, it has been known that the application of heat in the corneal stroma produces shrinkage of collagen.[1] In 1975 Gasset and Kaufman proposed thermokeratoplasty to correct the topographic abnormalities of keratoconus.[2] Keats and Dingle published that the initial flattening was followed by regression to pretreatment keratometric readings in seven of nine treated eyes.[3] Aquavella and his colleagues published many complications related to this technique only one year later, such as recurrent epithelial erosions and delayed healing, stromal necrosis melting and scarring, vascularization and fibrinous iritis with hypopyon.[4] The use of conventional thermal techniques up to that time was generated by a conductive heating method. Rowsey et al. proposed a new heating technique, the Los Alamos Thermokeratoplasty.[5]

Fyodorov in Moscow developed the radial thermokeratoplasty for the reduction of hyperopia.[6] In this technique, controlled thermal burns of the corneal stroma (with a retractable probe tip preset to penetrate the cornea at 95% depth) was used. A progressive decrease in the initial correction was noticed and the procedure has been gradually abandoned.[7,8]

In April 1993, we found that high-frequency, low-energy current applied with a probe which touched the surface of the cornea—when applied in a series of eight spots of one millimeter in diameter distributed symmetrically around a seven millimeter diameter ring in the mid-periphery of the cornea—produced steeping which corrected hyperopia. This hyperopic correction was stable and had little regression through time.

PATIENT SELECTION

With a retrospective view of our first 166 cases from April 1993 to September 1994 we found that our best candidates were patients over 35 years of age, with keratometry readings under 4.00 D, and central pachymetry of under 550 microns with a hyperopia of +3.50 Diopters (D) or less.

ENERGY ABSORPTION

We also learned that we need the energy concentrated in a small spot, the deeper in the corneal stroma the better. Tear film or balanced salt solution (BSS) on the corneal surface dissipate the energy superficially and restrict penetration. This was the reason for regression in some cases. Bowman's layer also absorbed a greater part of the energy—making the spot wider and preventing good penetration. With the superficial application of high frequency current we needed an output energy of 3 joules (J) for 1 second, reaching 85% depth of the mid periphery cornea. The application of the energy directly to the stroma was very important. This way less energy is required in achieving the same amount of effect.

CURRENT EQUIPMENT

The Mendez Corneal Shaper (MCS™) consists of a console containing the energy delivery system controlled by a digital timer. This device is activated by a foot pedal connected to the back panel. On the front panel there is an energy output adjustment and a digital timer, both may be controlled manually by the surgeon. Two connections are also present for the leads of the wire speculum and the handpiece. The wire speculum and the keratoplast™ tips must be sterile before use.

When we started applying the energy with the intrastromal technique, even better patient results were accomplished. This technique is referred to as intrastromal conductive keratoplasty (IRK).

Intrastromal application of high frequency current is done through a very fine tip that measures 400 microns in length and 100 microns in diameter (Fig. 17–1). The base of the tip is insulated to prevent loss of current through tear film, epithelium and the greater part of Bowman's layer. The length of the tip varies depending on the central pachymetry of the patient's cornea (Table 17–1). Because of the characteristics of the delicate Keratoplast™ tip, we have found more consistent results using a new tip per case.

With this tip we have measured an energy output of 0.5 J in 0.75 seconds. This reduces the size of the residual leukoma significantly while maintaining the effect. Measuring the temperature is difficult, collagen fibers need between 50° and 60°C to contract without necrosis.

CURRENT SURGICAL TECHNIQUE

A complete ophthalmologic exam is necessary before treating any patient. This includes visual acuity, best corrected visual acuity, refraction, refraction under cycloplegia, keratometry, biomicroscopy with slit lamp, tonometry, central ultrasonic pachymetry, computer assisted videokeratoscopy, and fundoscopic examination.

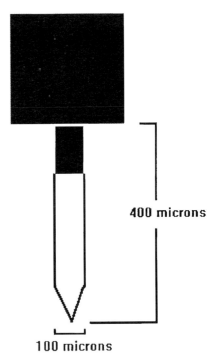

400 microns

100 microns

Fig. 17–1. Intrastromal application of high frequency current is done through a very fine tip that measures 400 microns in length and 100 microns in diameter.

The procedure is explained to the patient preoperatively and it is very important to advise the patient that for the first few weeks, he or she will have a myopic effect. This is normal because at first the patient is overcorrected, allowing for the predetermined amount of regression to take effect.

On the date the procedure is scheduled, the patient is premedicated with 5mg of Valium 30 minutes before the procedure. The patient is positioned under an operating microscope. Topical proparacaine is used, the grounded lid speculum is placed and the patient is asked to stare at a fixating light

Table 17–1. Tip Selection

Central Corneal Pachymetry	Length of Tip to be Used
500 to 549 microns	400 microns
550 or greater	450 microns

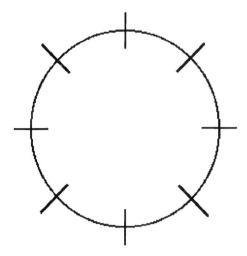

Fig. 17–2. The MCKM consist of a 6mm or 7mm optical zone mark with eight symmetrical intersections of 1mm.

under the microscope. The visual axis is determined and an inked Mendez conductive keratoplasty marker (MCKM) used over the cornea. The MCKM consist of a 6mm or 7mm optical zone mark with eight symmetrical intersections of 1mm (Fig. 17–2).

There is no need to fixate the globe. The patient is asked to stare at a fixating light and the sterile Keratoplast™ tip is placed in the intersection of the straight line and the optical zone mark. The tip pen-

etrates easily without much pressure. The tip penetration is precalibrated by an insulated mechanical stop. Once proper penetration is achieved, the foot pedal of the MCS is activated delivering the energy to the deeper corneal layers. The same procedure is repeated until the complete treatment is accomplished.

The denatured epithelium is removed to facilitate epithelium migration, antibiotic drops (tobramicin) are instilled and the speculum is removed. The amount of spots per case is determined by the amount of correction desired. (Table 17–2, Figures 17–3, 17–4, and 17–5). Our current technique allows the power and time settings to remain unchanged. If astigmatism is present, greater amount of treatment will be needed in the flatter meridians to induce steepening in this area.

Once the full treatment is applied, the patient may be taken to the auto refractor to analyze the results. Depending on the epithelium drying and edema, the patient may be able to have very good near vision immediately.

The patient is managed postoperatively with topical antibiotics (Tobramicin) involving two drops every two hours for 24 hours, then every eight hours for five days, Diclofenac sodium every eight hours for two days, and oral analgesic for 24 hours. The epithelium heals in 48 to 72 hours. The patient is seen at 24 hours, two days, one week, two weeks, one month, three months, six months and one year postop.

Table 17–2. Nomogram, Energy Setting at 10, Time Setting at 0.75 Sec.

Refraction	Number of Spots	Number of Rows	Optical Zone	Immediate Post Op Refraction
+1.00 D to +1.50 D	16	2	7 mm, 8 mm	−1.50 D
+2.00 D to +2.50 D	24	3	6 mm, 7 mm 8 mm	−2.00 D
+3.00 D to +3.50 D	32	4	6 mm, 7 mm 8 mm	−2.00 D

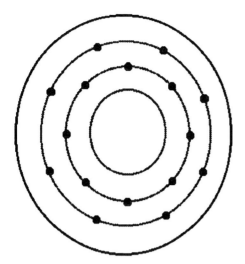

Fig. 17–3. Pattern of application of energy for the correction of +1.00 D to +1.50 D.

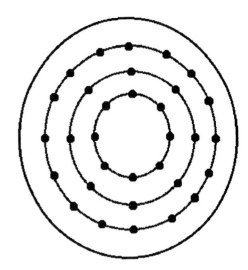

Fig. 17–5. Pattern of application of energy for the correction of +3.00 D to +3.50 D.

CURRENT RESULTS

Sixty-seven eyes of 34 patients from October 1994 to February 1996 underwent the procedure. Eleven patients were male and 23 female. Age ranged from 30 to 65 years. See Table 17–3 for age breakdown. To date, there is postoperative follow-up of one to sixteen months with 67 patients who were treated with the ICK technique.

Spherical equivalent with cycloplegic preoperative refraction ranged from +1.50 to +5.50. Most of the patients were between +2.50 D and +3.50 D (Table 17–4).

The immediate postop refraction in patients ranges from −1.50 D to −2.50 D, which decrease to −1.00 D in three to six months (Table 17–5 and 17–6), and reach plano at one year (Table 17–7).

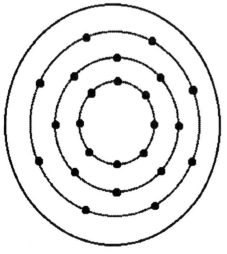

Fig. 17–4. Pattern of application of energy for the correction of +2.00 D to +2.50 D.

Table 17–3. Age Distribution

Number of Patients	Range of Age
5 (15%)	20 to 40 years
11 (32%)	41 to 50 years
17 (50%)	51 to 60 years
1 (3%)	61 to 65 years

Table 17.4. Preoperative Refraction and Number of Cases (67 Eyes)

Pre-op Refraction	Number of Patients
+1.50 D	12 eyes (18%)
+2.00 D	8 eyes (12%)
+2.50 D	16 eyes (24%)
+3.00 D	10 eyes (16%)
+3.50 D	9 eyes (13%)
+4.00 D	5 eyes (8%)
+4.50 D	3 eyes (4%)
+5.00 D	1 eye (1%)
+5.50 D	3 eyes (4%)

Table 17.7. Postoperative Refraction and Number of Cases at 12 months (20 Eyes)

Post-op Refraction at 12 Months	Number of Eyes
−0.50 D	5 eyes (25%)
Plano	2 eyes (10%)
+0.50 D	3 eyes (15%)
+1.00 D	8 eyes (40%)
+1.50 D	1 eye (5%)
+2.00 D	1 eye (5%)

Table 17.5. Postoperative Refraction and Number of Cases at 1 to 3 Months (67 Eyes)

Post-op Refraction at 1 to 3 months	Number of Eyes
−2.00 D	6 eyes (9%)
−1.50 D	12 eyes (18%)
−1.00 D	15 eyes (22%)
−0.50 D	10 eyes (15%)
Plano	9 eyes (13%)
+0.50 D	11 eyes (17%)
+1.50 D	2 eyes (3%)
+3.00 D	2 eyes (3%)

During this time, the patients may require visual aid with glasses for far vision.

Preoperative visual acuity in approximately half the patients (55%) ranged from 20/100 to 20/400. This is due to the low accommodation capabilities of patients over 40 years of age (Table 17–8). Postop visual acuity increased in all patients. Although, at three months, most patients are overcorrected. Visual acuity ranged from 20/20 to 20/30 in 60% of these cases (Table 17–9). Ninety-five percent of the patients reach the same range at six months (Table 17–10A). And of the 20 patients with one year postop, all except one range from 20/20 to 20/30 (Table 17–10B). Preop and postop results in the 20 cases of one year follow-up are shown in Tables 17–11 and 17–12.

Table 17.6. Postoperative Refraction and Number of Cases at 6 Months (44 Eyes)

Post-op Refraction at 6 months	Number of Eyes
−1.00 D	2 eyes
−0.50 D	10 eyes
Plano	9 eyes
+0.50 D	11 eyes
+1.00 D	10 eyes
+1.50 D	1 eye
+2.50 D	1 eye

Table 17.8. Preoperative Visual Acuity and Number of Eyes

Pre-op Visual Acuity	Number of Eyes
20/50	20 eyes (30%)
20/60	12 eyes (18%)
20/70	18 eyes (27%)
20/80	11 eyes (17%)
20/100	4 eyes (6%)
20/200	1 eye (1%)
20/400	1 eye (1%)

Table 17.9. Postoperative Visual Acuity and Number of Eyes at 1 to 3 Months (67 Eyes)

Post-op Visual Acuity 1 to 3 months	Number of Eyes
20/20	20 eyes (30%)
20/25	12 eyes (18%)
20/30	18 eyes (27%)
20/40	11 eyes (17%)
20/50	4 eyes (6%)
20/60	1 eye (1%)
20/70	1 eye (1%)

Table 17.10A. Postoperative Visual Acuity and Number of Eyes at 6 Months (44 Eyes)

Post-op Visual Acuity 6 Months	Number of Eyes
20/20	25 eyes
20/30	18 eyes
2070	1 eye

Table 17.10B. Postoperative Visual Acuity and Number of Eyes at 6 Months (44 eyes)

Post-op Visual Acuity 12 Months	Number of Eyes
20/20	13 eyes
20/30	6 eyes
20/70	1 eye

Slit lamp microscopy showed striae which run between each treatment spot forming a belt that contracts and steepens the central cornea (Figures 17–6 and 17–7). Keratometry readings also increased from 2 D to 5 D, depending on the amount of correction.

Table 17.11. Preoperative and 12 Month Postoperative Refraction of 20 Cases

Case	Pre Op Refraction	3 Months Post Op	6 Months Post Op	12 Months Post Op
1	.+4.00 D	.+1.50 D	.+1.50 D	.+1.00 D
2	.+3.50 D	.+1.00 D	.+1.00 D	.+1.00 D
3	.+2.00 D	.+0.50 D	.+0.50 D	.−0.50 D
4	.+1.50 D	.−0.50 D	.+0.50 D	.−0.50 D
5	.+4.50 D	.+0.50 D	.−0.50 D	.−0.50 D
6	.+5.50 D	.+2.00 D	.+2.50 D	.+2.00 D
7	.+5.50 D	.+1.50 D	.+1.00 D	.+1.00 D
8	.+5.50 D	.+1.50 D	.+1.00 D	.+1.00 D
9	.+3.50 D	.−1.50 D	.−1.00 D	.−.050 D
10	.+3.50 D	.−1.50 D	.−1.00 D	.−.050 D
11	.+4.00 D	.−1.00 D	.−0.50 D	.+0.50 D
12	.+4.50 D	.−1.50 D	.−0.50 D	.+1.50 D
13	.+3.50 D	.−1.00 D		.+0.50 D
14	.+3.50 D	.−1.00 D		.+0.50 D
15	.+3.50 D	.−0.50 D		.+1.00 D
16	.+4.00 D	.−0.50 D		.+1.00 D
17	.+3.50 D	.+0.50 D	.+0.75 D	.+1.00 D
18	.+3.50 D	.+0.50 D	.+0.75 D	.+1.00 D
19	.+2.50 D	PLANO	.−0.50 D	PLANO
20	.+2.50 D	PLANO	.−0.50 D	PLANO

Table 17.12. Preoperative and 12 Month Postoperative Visual Acuity of 20 Cases

Case	Preop V.A.	3 Months Post Op V.A.	6 Months Post Op V.A.	12 Months Pos Op V.A.
1	20/200	20/25	20/30	20/30
2	20/200	20/30	20/25	20/25
3	20/50	20/20	20/20	20/20
4	20/50	20/20	20/20	20/20
5	20/200	20/20	20/20	20/20
6	20/400	20/200	20/70	20/70
7	20/400	20/30	20/25	20/25
8	20/400	20/30	20/25	20/25
9	20/60	20/20	20/20	20/20
10	20/60	20/20	20/20	20/20
11	20/100	20/30	20/25	20/20
12	20/80	20/30	20/25	20/20
13	20/100	20/25	20/25	20/20
14	20/100	20/25	20/25	20/20
15	20/200	20/25	20/20	20/20
16	20/400	20/25	20/20	20/20
17	20/200	20/20	20/20	20/25
18	20/400	20/20	20/20	20/25
19	20/200	20/20	20/20	20/20
20	20/200	20/20	20/20	20/20

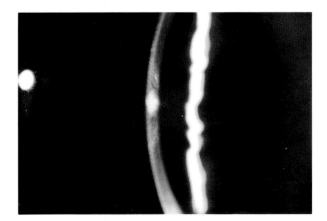

Fig. 17–6. Slit lamp microscopy showed striae which run between each treatment spot forming a belt that contracts and steepens the central cornea. Keratometry readings also increased from 2 D to 5 D, depending on the amount of correction.

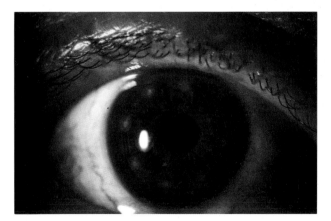

Fig. 17–7. Treatment pattern immediate postop.

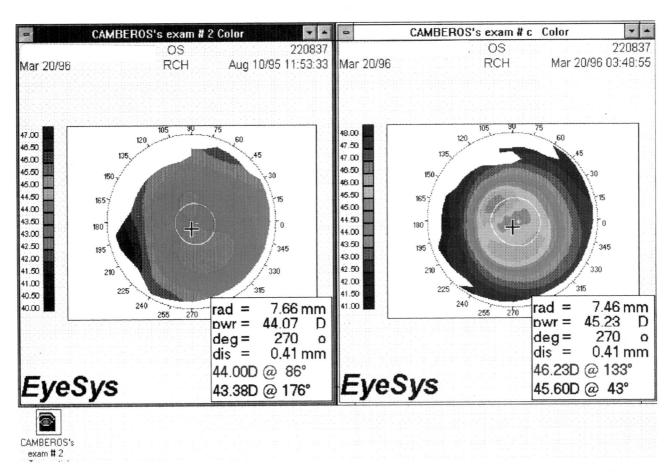

Fig. 17–8. Computer assisted video topography shows a steepened area in the center of the cornea with a diameter in the tangential map of the EyeSys™ video topography of 3.5mm surrounded by an area of corneal flattening.

Figure 17–8 is a computer assisted video topography which shows a steepened area in the center of the cornea with a diameter in the tangential map of the EyeSys™ video topography of 3.5mm surrounded by an area of corneal flattening.

HISTOLOGY

A report by Marcia Reis Guimaraes, M.D., Ricardo Guimaraes M.D., Ph.D., and Raul Damásio Castro, M.D. on a short-term histopathologic analysis of six human cornea that had radio-frequency current applied using the Mendez Corneal Shaping System (MCS™), found thermal injury to the epithelium, an intact Bowman membrane with discrete shrink-

age of its fibers, and a shrunken and edematous stroma.[9] Discrete injury to Descemet's membrane and endothelial cells was found in only two out of six cases. No severe necrosis or inflammatory cells were present indicating the technique gives more stable results.

COMPLICATIONS

Induced irregular astigmatism may be present when the application of the high frequency current is not done symmetrically on the entire treatment. Retreatment may be performed safely at the slit lamp. We have not seen any case of recurrent erosion or infection.

FUTURE PLANS AND DEVELOPMENT

Although this equipment is not yet on the market and is still being used on an experimental basis, research is still being done to make this procedure even more efficient. Many developments are underway which will enhance the intrastromal conductive keratoplasty procedure.

REFERENCES

1. Lans LJ: Experimentelle untersuchnger uber die entstehung von astigmatismus duch nich-perforierende corneawunden. *Albrecht von Graefes Arch Klin Exper Ophthalmol* 1898:117–152.
2. Gasset AR, Kaufman HE: Thermokeratoplasty in the treatment of keratoconus. *Am J Ophthalmol* 79:226–232, 1975.
3. Keats RH, Dingle J: Thermokeratoplasty for keratoconus. *Ophthalmic Surg* 6(3):89–92, 1975.
4. Aquavella JV, Smith RS, Shaw EL: Alterations in corneal morphology following thermokeratoplasty. *Arch Ophthalmol* 94:2082–2085, 1976.
5. Rowsey JJ: Electrosurgical Keratoplasty: Update and retraction. *Invest Ophthalmol Vis Sci.* ARVO Abstracts 28(suppl):224, 1987.
6. Newmann AC, Fyodorov S, Sander DR: Radial thermokeratoplasty for the correction of hyperopia. *Refract Corneal Surg* 6:404–412, 1990.
7. Newman AC, Sander DR, Raanan M, DeLuca M: Hyperopic thermokeratoplasty: Clinical evaluation. *J Cataract Refract Surg* 17:830–838, 1991.
8. Feldman ST, Ellis W, Frucht-Pery J, et al: Regression of effect following radial thermokeratoplasty in humans. *Refract Corneal Surg* 5:288–291, 1989.
9. Guimaraes MR, Guimaraes RQ, Castro RD: Symposium on Cataract, IOL and Refractive Surgery. San Diego, CA. April 1995.

section VI
Implants

CHAPTER 18

Clear Lens Extraction with Intraocular Lens Implantation for the Correction of Hyperopia

Amir H. K. Isfahani
James Salz

INTRODUCTION

Over the past twenty-five years refractive surgery has been primarily devoted to the correction of myopia and astigmatism, by modifying corneal curvature. There is now more evidence that hyperopia is actually more common than myopia and hence, there is an increasing interest in the surgical correction of hyperopia. A large number of surgical procedures for the treatment of hyperopia have been proposed, but their use has been met with limited success.

CLASSIFICATION OF HYPEROPIA

Hyperopia can be classified as mild (0.00 to +6.00), moderate (+6.00 to +10.00) or high (>+10.00). Currently the surgical procedures available for mild hyperopia include holmium laser thermokeratoplasty, excimer photorefractive keratectomy (PRK) and automated lamellar keratectomy (ALK) (Table 18–1). Holmium laser thermokeratoplasty has been used for the correction of hyperopia in the range of +1.00 to +5.00 diopters (D) but regression has been the limiting factor with its use within this range.[1,2] Excimer laser photorefractive keratectomy can be used as an efficient and relatively safe procedure for the correction of hyperopia up to 7.5 D.[3] Relative success has also been reported with hyperopic automated lamellar keratoplasty for hyperopia up to +6.00 D.[4] Hexagonal keratotomy for correction of low hyperopia is no longer commonly used secondary to refractive instability and a high incidence of surgical induced irregular astigmatism.[5,6]

APHAKIA

The incidence of aphakic hyperopia has been steadily decreasing in recent years with the increased use of primary or secondary intraocular lens implantation that offers rapid and accurate visual recovery. However, the surgical correction of phakic moderate to high hyperopia still remains a challenging problem. The current surgical procedures available for moderate and high hyperopia are laser in-situ keratomileusis (LASIK), epikeratoplasty,[7,8] phakic intraocular lens, and clear lens extraction with intraocular lens (IOL).[9–12]

CLEAR LENS EXTRACTION

Clear lens extraction with IOL for correction of hyperopia has been recently described by Signanos.[8,9] They reported their results in seventeen normally sighted hyperopic eyes of nine patients which underwent extracapsular clear lens extraction and biconvex IOL implantation. Intraocular lens calculation was performed by the SRK II formula and IOL power was chosen for a postoperative refraction of −1.50 D. The mean spherical equivalent for distance was 9.61 D (range 6.75 to 13.75 D) with a mean uncorrected visual acuity of count fingers. Postoperatively, the mean spherical equivalent for distance was +0.06 D (range −0.37 to +0.50 D) with all eyes achieving an uncorrected visual acuity of 20/50 or better (range of 20/20–20/50 Snellen visual acuity). There was no loss of best spectacle corrected Snellen visual acuity in this group. The postoperative results were stable

Table 18–1. Surgical Methods of Correcting Hyperopia

Level of Hyperopia	Surgical Procedures
Mild	Holmium Thermokeratoplasty
	Eximer Photorefractive Keratectomy
	Automated Lamellar Keratoplasty
	Hexagonal Keratotomy (Not Recommended)
Moderate to High	Laser in situ Keratomileusis
	Epikeratoplasty
	Phakic Intraocular Lens
	Clear lens extraction with Intraocular lens

over the follow-up period of 1–3 years (mean follow-up of 26.2 months), and all the patients were satisfied with the results.

It should be noted that Signanos reported a discrepancy between the intended postoperative refraction of −1.50 D using the SRK II formula and the actual mean postoperative refractive equivalent of +0.06 D. Using the Hoffer Q formula, we observed an IOL error margin of +0.74 diopters compared to Signanos's reported IOL error margin of +1.56 diopters using the SRK II formula.

CURRENT SURGICAL TECHNIQUE AND CLINICAL RESULTS

We have also been encouraged by our own clinical experience with clear lens extraction with IOL in sixteen hyperopic eyes of nine patients. Their demographic and clinical data is presented in Tables 18–2 and 18–3. All patients underwent extracapsular clear lens extraction using phacoemulsification technique and capsular bag biconvex IOL implantation. Intraocular lens calculation was performed using the Hoffer Q formula. Preoperatively, the mean spherical equivalent for distance was +5.86 D (range of +4.25 to +9.625 D). Postoperatively, the mean spherical equivalent for distance was −0.16 D (range of −2.50 to +1.375 D) with all eyes achieving an uncorrected visual acuity of 20/50 or better (range of 20/30–20/50 Snellen visual acuity).

Lyle et al.[11] have also reported encouraging results with clear lens extraction in six hyperopic eyes. All patients underwent phacoemulsification

Table 18–2. Preoperative Patient Data

Age, Sex	Pre-Op BCVA	Pre-Op Refraction	Axial length
1/F/65	20/50	+5.25	21.31
2/F/65	20/20	+5.25 − 1.25 × 65	21.51
1/M/49	20/30	+5.50 − 0.50 × 30	22.65
2/M/49	20/20	+4.75 − 0.25 × 20	22.62
1/M/50	20/25	+8.50 − 4.50 × 93	21.35
2/M/50	20/25	+6.50 − 2.75 × 68	21.75
1/M/44	20/20	+8.00 − 1.75 × 110	20.03
2/M/44	20/20	+7.75 − 1.75 × 48	20.08
1/F/67	20/40	+10.00 − 0.75 × 10	21.21
2/F/67	20/40	+9.75 − 0.75 × 10	21.47
1/F/55	20/40	+4.50	21.66
1/F/65	20/40	+5.50 − 2.00 × 005	21.62
2/F/65	20/30	+7.50 − 2.00 × 175	20.98
1/M/69	20/40	+5.25 − 0.75 × 84	22.84
1/M/51	20/20	+5.25 − 0.50 × 80	20.72
2/M/51	20/20	+5.25 − 1.00 × 170	20.69

Table 18–3. Postoperative Data

UCVA	Post-Op BCVA	Post-Op Refraction	IOL Error	Follow-up
20/50	20/30	+1.00 − 0.25 × 90	+0.375	3 months
20/40	20/30	plano − 1.50 × 45	+0.25	3 months
20/30	20/25	+0.50 − 0.50 × 180	+0.75	12 months
20/40	20/30	+1.00 − 0.75 × 180	+1.625	10 months
20/50	20/30	+1.75 − 2.00 × 95	+1.75	6 months
20/50	20/25	+2.00 − 2.00 × 75	+2.00	6 months
20/30	20/20	plano − 2.00 × 107	+2.00	9 months
20/30	20/20	plano − 1.00 × 47	+1.50	9 months
20/50	20/30	−1.00 − 0.75 × 180	+1.125	8 months
20/40	20/30	−1.00 − 1.00 × 180	+0.50	8 months
20/30	20/20	+1.25	+1.25	2 months
20/30	20/20	+0.25 − 1.00 × 90	−0.25	24 months
20/40	20/20	+0.25 − 0.75 × 90	−0.125	14 months
20/50	20/20	+2.00 − 1.25 × 90	+1.375	12 months
20/40	20/20	−0.25 − 1.00 × 120	−0.75	2 months
20/40	20/20	−2.25 − 0.50 × 90	−1.50	2 months

and capsular bag IOL implantation using the SRK II formula. The mean preoperative spherical equivalent was +6.52 D (range of +4.25 to +7.87) and the mean postoperative spherical equivalent was −0.42 D (range of −0.75 to +0.87). All six hyperopic eyes achieved a postoperative visual acuity of 20/40 or better.

The clinical data for these three series is summarized in Table 18–4. A total of thirty-nine hyperopic eyes underwent clear lens extraction with IOL implantation. Overall, the mean preoperative spherical equivalent was +7.33 D and the mean postoperative spherical equivalent was −0.01 D. All eyes achieved an uncorrected visual acuity of 20/50 or better.

Patients with moderate to high hyperopia are truly disabled without optical correction since they can not see at near or distance. This becomes an increasing problem with advancing age towards presbyopia because it requires addition of more plus diopters to the already existing plus correction. This will in turn lead to further spherical and chromatic aberration with consequent reduction in image quality. We believe the results of clear lens extraction with IOL in these 39 hyperopic eyes clearly support that this is an excellent surgical option in the age group of 35 or older.

Table 18–4. Summary of Ascan and Biometry

Number of eyes	39
Age	
mean	49.3 years
Range	35–69 years
Axial Lengths	
mean	20.71 mm
Range	17.88–22.78 mm
Pre-op Refraction (SE)	
mean	+7.33 diopters
range	+4.25 to +13.75 diopters
Post-op Refraction (SE)	
mean	−0.01 diopters
range	−2.50 to +1.375 diopters
IOL error margin	
SRK II	+1.04 diopters
Hoffer Q	+0.74 diopters
Follow-up	
mean	17.78 months
range	2–36 months

In the age group of 35 years or younger, there is a dilemma involving clear lens extraction with IOL, since this surgical procedure would then deprive the patients of their natural accommodative power.

With further refinement, more reliable and accurate IOL formulas for these hyperopic eyes will be developed and clear lensectomy with IOL could then be recommended in this age group. Phakic posterior chamber intraocular lens implantation is also an attractive option in these younger patients allowing them to retain their accommodation.

COMPLICATIONS

In this combined series of 39 eyes which underwent clear lens extraction with IOL implantation, there were no cases of retinal detachment, cystoid macular edema, endophthalmitis, suprachoroidal hemorrhage, uveal effusion or malignant glaucoma, surgical induced irregular astigmatism or loss of best corrected visual acuity. Several complications have been reported. Complications associated with this surgical procedure are similar to those reported with cataract extraction and IOL. The most common intraoperative complication of capsular rupture and vitreous loss has been reported in one case. Another frequent complication is posterior capsule opacification (PCO) that has been reported in three cases (18%) with an average opacification time of 20 months. In this younger patient population one might have expected a higher rate of PCO compared to the older patients who routinely undergo cataract extraction with IOL. However, it appears that the rate of PCO is lower or at the same rate as the older patients. All three patients underwent successful Nd-YAG capsulotomy with no complications such as cystoid macula edema or retinal detachment.

Signanos has also evaluated the potential long-term complication of corneal decompensation and have reported mean endothelial cell loss of 10% with their extracapsular lens extraction technique. This endothelial cell loss was found to be stable over the follow-up period of 3 years. Their reported endothelial cell loss was relatively high but with modern phacoemulsification technique, the endothelial loss should be much lower. There was an observed surgically induced regular astigmatism of 0.5 to 2.00 diopters. This is very similar to the induced astigmatism after cataract surgery and the surgical wound incision should be adjusted according to the cornea astigmatism to optimize postoperative refraction.

NANOPHTHALMOS

Nanophthalmos is a rare disorder with characteristic features of a small eye and a small cornea, a shallow anterior chamber, moderate to high hyperopia, short axial length of less than 20.5 mm and diffuse choroidal-scleral thickening.[13,14] Intraocular surgery on nanophthalmic eyes increases the possibility of both intraoperative and postoperative complications, and surgery on these eyes should be approached with great caution and full disclosure of the potential risks. Although uveal effusion may occur spontaneously in nanophthalmic eyes, massive uveal effusion, retinal detachment, intraocular hemorrhage and malignant glaucoma can all occur in these eyes after cataract surgery. In the event of intraoperative or postoperative massive choroidal effusion, sclerectomy or unsutured sclerotomy as recommended by Anderson[14] can be considered for the management of this complication.

IMPLANTATION IN AN NANOPHTHALMIC EYE

Recently we have performed clear lens extraction with implantation of two biconvex IOL's in a nanophthalmic eye which was complicated by inaccurate IOL power calculation most likely due to the fact that the anterior lens (+12.00) was inadvertently placed in the sulcus, rather than in the bag with the posterior lens (+34.00). The details of this case are summarized as follows:

Preoperative data: VAsc 20/400 ou, OD +9.00 −1.00 × 175 = 20/20, OS +9.25 −0.75 × 170 = 20/20. Keratometry OD 48.25/50.25, OS 48.50/50.00, Ta 15 mmHG ou. Corneal diameter 10.50 mm ou. Immersion A scan OD 17.71 mm, OS 17.64 mm, AC depth OD 2.73 mm, OS 2.83 mm, Lens thickness OD 4.77 mm, OS 4.66 mm.

Formulas: Hoffer OD +46.00 = −1.54 D, OS +47.00 = −1.75 D with A constant 119.0.

Holladay OD +44.50 = −1.00 D, OS +45.00 = −1.00 D with A constant 119.0.

Lenses implanted OS posterior +34.00 D with anterior +12.00 D, Alcon MC60BM with A constant of 119.0.

At surgery, pupil became somewhat miotic and with relatively small anterior capsulorhexis, the anterior IOL was inadvertently placed in the sulcus rather than in the bag.

Post-Operative Course:

POD # 1. VAsc 20/70, manifest ref −0.50 −1.50 × 180 = 20/30 with deep AC and mid-dilated pupil. Ta = 16.

POD # 6. VAsc 20/400, manifest ref −5.00 −1.50 × 15 = 20/40 with very shallow AC with an IOP of 20.

Two YAG peripheral iridotomies were performed without difficulty but the AC remained shallow. The possibilities for the refractive change include choroidal effusion (none were seen on indirect exam) and anterior movement of both IOL's during the postoperative period. This may have been the result of the cycloplegia and also due to lack of pressure on the posterior IOL since the anterior IOL was in the sulcus rather than in the capsular bag. Treatment included 1% prednisolone q 2h and Timoptic XE qd.

POD #10. VAsc 20/400, manifest ref −6.00 −1.00 × 180 = 20/40, with shallow AC and patent PI's

POD #14. B scan of posterior segment revealed no choroidal and diffuse choroidal-scleral thickening. Patient noted vision improvement with cycloplegia during retinal exam. Treatment included 1% prednisolone q 4h and Homatropine tid.

POD #16. B scan of anterior segment by Dr. Barry Kerman of the Jules Stein Eye Institute, revealed no anterior choroidals, normal ciliary body and two IOL's noted on top of each other with minimal tilt and 1.0 mm decentration of the anterior IOL (Fig. 18–1). POD #16 (pt was still on Homatropine drops) VAsc 20/100 manifest ref −2.50 −1.00 × 180 = 20/30, Homatropine was discontinued so that the natural AC depth, lens position and refraction can be determined.

POD #21. VAsc 20/400 with manifest ref −6.50 = 20/30. Surgical options considered were RK, IOL exchange

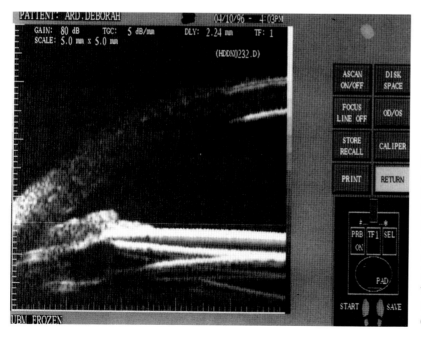

Fig. 18–1. Anterior segment B-scan with ultrasound biomicroscopy. (Humphrey instrument) demonstrating the 2 biconvex intraocular lenses. The anterior lens is slightly tilted and is displacing the iris anteriorly. There was no ciliary body effusion. At surgery to exchange the anterior lens, one loop was in the sulcus and one loop was in the capsular bag. (Photo courtesy of Dr. Barry Kerman at UCLA Department of Ophthalmology)

with consultation with Dr. Holladay for IOL power of the replacement lens in the sulcus.

POD #23. The patient opted for an IOL exchange. During the surgery one of the haptic of the anterior IOL was noted to be in the bag and the other in the sulcus. The anterior IOL was dialed out of the bag and the a +6.00 D Alcon MC60BM with A constant of 119.0 was placed in the sulcus. Dr. Holladay calculated the IOL power for intended postoperative scan of anterior segment by Dr. Barry Kerman of the Jules Stein Eye Institute, revealed no anterior choroidals, normal ciliary body and two IOL's noted on top of each other with minimal tilt and 1.0 mm decentration of the anterior IOL (Fig. 18.1). refractive error of −1.50.

POD #24. VAsc 20/80 with manifest ref of −0.75 −2.00 × 180 = 20/40. The patient was maintained on cycloplegia for four days post IOL exchange.

POD #29. pt presented with marked anterior displacement of both IOL's with central anterior chamber and flat peripheral anterior chamber, with an IOP of 18. Indirect ophthalmoscopy revealed no choroidal effusion. It was felt that there was most likely misdirection of aqueous posteriorly pushing the vitreous and the capsule bag anteriorly. The eye was dilated with homatropine 5% tid.

POD #30. VAsc was 20/80 with manifest ref −0.75 −2.00 × 180 = 20/40. She will be maintained on homatropine for the next two weeks and if the chamber again shallows on cessation of the homatropine, YAG laser capsulotomy and UAG laser opening in the vitreous face will be performed in an attempt to re-establish normal aqueous dynamics. In case this laser surgical intervention fails, then either medical management with long-term cycloplegia or possible pars plana vit-

rectomy will be considered. She has again been encouraged to attempt contact lens fitting in her other eye in order to avoid clear lens extraction of her other eye.

IOL CALCULATIONS PROBLEMS

The limiting factor in improving the success of clear lens extraction with IOL in hyperopic eyes is the relative inaccuracy of modern IOL calculation formulas. Signanos has reported an IOL error margin of approximately +1.5 diopters and in our clinical experience with the Hoffer Q formula, we observe an IOL error margin of approximately +0.75 diopters. Current third generation formulas (Holladay, SRK/T and Hoffer Q) are better than older formulas for extremely short eyes, but still are not acceptable for the desired clinical accuracy.[15] Holladay has pointed out that short eyes can have either small, normal or large anterior segments and it is thought that this variation in the size of the anterior segment that accounts for the inaccuracy expected with available IOL calculation formulas. Currently Holladay is developing a more advanced formula which takes into account anterior segment measurements such as corneal diameter, anterior chamber depth and lens thickness. We expect this new formula to be more accurate and should be available for commercial use in the near future.

Although in each of the reported 39 eyes, single biconvex IOL was used since IOL powers of up to 34.00 diopters are commercially available. Increasing spherical aberration is the main reason that IOL power of greater than 35.00 diopters are not manufactured and capsular bag piggy-back lenses are recommended. Some have recommended using two plano-convex IOLs with two plano sides on top of each other to prevent decentration. However Holladay[15] recommended two piggy-back biconvex lens with their optical-center aligned within the capsular bag. He believes that this results in superior optical quality with less spherical aberration.

SUMMARY

Clear lens extraction with IOL to correct moderate to high hyperopia is an efficient, safe and predictable surgical procedure. We believe that in patients 35 years or older, clear lensectomy with IOL is superior to other surgical techniques for the correction of moderate to high hyperopia. Furthermore, echography should be used to diagnose and prevent inadvertent surgery on nanophthalmic eyes since these eyes are at great risk for post-operative complications. With further refinement of IOL calculation formulas for these small eyes, clear lensectomy with IOL implantation will become more accurate and predictable.

REFERENCES

1. Moriera H, Campos M, Sawusch MR et al: Holmium laser thermokeratoplasty. *Ophthalmology* 100:752–761, 1993.
2. Ariyasu RG, Sand B, Menefee R et al: Holmium laser thermal keratoplasty of 10 poorly sighted eyes. *J Refract Surg* 11:3580–3565, 1995.
3. Dausch D, Klein R, Schroder E: Excimer laser photorefractive keratectomy for hyperopia. *Refract Corneal Surg* 9:20–28, 1993.
4. Manche EE, Judge A, Maloney RK: Lamellar keratoplasty for hyperopia. *J Refract Surg* 12:42–49, 1996.
5. Neuman AC, McCarty GR: Hexagonal keratotomy for correction of low hyperopia: preliminary results of a prospective study. *J Cataract Refract Surg* 14:265–269, 1988.
6. Casebeer JC, Phillips SG: Hexagonal keratotomy. A historical review and assessment of 46 cases. *Ophth Clin North Am* 5:727–744, 1992.
7. Ehrlich MI, Nordan LT: Epikeratophakia for the treatment of hyperopia. *J Cataract Refract Surg* 15:661–666, 1989.
8. McDonald MB, Kaufman HE, Aquavella JV et al: The nationwide study of epikeratiphakia for aphakia in adults. *AJO* 103:358–365, 1987.
9. Siganos DS, Siganos CS, Pallikaris IG: Clear lens extraction and intraocular lens implantation in normally sighted hyperopic eyes. *J Refract Corneal Surg* 10:117–24, 1994.
10. Siganos DS, Pallikaris IG, Siganos CS: Clear lensectomy and intraocular lens implantation in normally sighted highly hyperopic eyes. Three-year follow-up. *Eur J Implant Ref Surg* 7:128–133, 1995.
11. Lyle WA, Jin GJC: Clear lens extraction for the correction of high refractive error. *J Cataract Refract Surg* 20:273–276, 1994.
12. Ostbaum SA: Clear lens extraction for myopia and high hyperopia. *J Cataract Refract Surg* 20:271, 1994.
13. Byrne SF, Green RL: *Ultrasound of the Eye and Orbit,* St. Louis, Mosby-Year book, 1992, pp 240–243.
14. Jin JC, Anderson DR: Laser and unsutured sclerotomy in nanophthalmos. *Am J Ophthalmal* 109:575–580, 1990.
15. Holladay JT, Gills JP, Leidlein J et al: Achieving emmetropia in extremely short eyes with two piggyback posterior chamber lenses. Submitted for Publication.

CHAPTER 19

Phakic Intraocular Lens Implantation for Hyperopia

Daljit Singh

INTRODUCTION

Hypermetropia, especially high hypermetropia is a sight threatening condition in some children. In our daily clinical practice, we find that amblyopia is very common among hypermetropes, especially in cases of anisometropia. If the use of corrective glasses is not started at an early age, the chances of strabismus and amblyopia increase. Corrected visual acuity in hypermetropes is often diminished. Besides amblyopia, high hypermetropes suffer from all those problems that are to be found in aphakes using high plus power aphakic glasses. High hypermetropes have poor near vision, therefore they find it difficult to manage contact lenses.

Personal Historical Review

In 1985, I performed ECCE with high power iris-claw lens to improve the sight of 4 hypermetropic amblyopes. Each one of them felt better than before. However, to my mind there were a number of objections in this approach. They were:

1. It was difficult to get intraocular lens powers more than +28.
2. There was further need for the management of secondary cataract and all the possible problems of aphakic cum pseudophakic eyes.
3. In case a good eye were to be operated upon, there will be a loss of accommodation.

Keeping these objections in mind, it was considered appropriate to try plus power intraocular lenses in phakic high hypermetropes.

Intraocular Lens Selection

There are two types of intraocular lenses made for this purpose: an angle supported lens and an iris supported lens. An angle-supported lens was perceived to be hazardous. The problems inherent in the angle support system include peripheral synechia formation, tissue erosion in the angle, progressive pupil ovalling, chronic inflammation, glaucoma and corneal decompensation.

The second option was the iris-support in the form of an iris-claw lens. The iris claw lens is totally unlike the pupil supported lenses of the past. These lenses are uniplanar in construction in contrast to the pupil supported lenses that are three dimensional. Iris-claw lenses are made from well known nonbiodegradable material, e.g., PMMA. An iris-claw lens bridges across the pupil without disturbing it, it is away from the angle and away from the corneal endothelium. At the time of the surgery, the centration of the optic of the lens is under the full control of the surgeon. Once fixed in place, the lens stays in the same position. I have performed over 6500 iris claw lenses in aphakic eyes between 1979 and 1986. These lenses are extremely well tolerated by the aphakic eyes. The option of atraumatic explantation was always available.

CRITERIA FOR PATIENT SELECTION

Attempts were made to select only those cases who were visually crippled as a result of high hypermetropia. Further, if a patient had one good eye and the other eye was amblyopic, the latter was selected for surgery (the idea being to improve the uncorrected visual acuity and the side vision for navigation). The better eye usually had lesser degree of refractive error and it was left untouched.

We started the plus power iris-claw lens implantation in 1986. In 1991, this procedure was stopped, when we acquired an excimer laser since there was a hope that hypermetropia may become treatable with the new modality. We have used excimer laser since 1993, but the results are below expectation and are not comparable to the results with phakic intraocular lenses. With the 7 mm ablation zone that we used, the recovery has been slow to come, and have been fairly unpredictable. Recently we have started sutureless lens implantation of iris-claw lenses in phakic hypermetropes. We have also started 9 mm PRK for hypermetropes. A comparison of the two new approaches will be available in due course of time.

The Lens Design

The design of an iris claw lens is well known. It has an optic and two ring like haptics, one on each side. A cut in the haptic ring converts the haptic into an iris catching device (the claw). The claw may be symmetrical (Worst), wherein the two sides of the claw are of same size, or asymmetrical (Singh), wherein the claws are of unequal size and consequently of different strength and elasticity. The longer claw is more flexible than the smaller claw. The optics of the lenses used in phakic hypermetropes are convexo-concave. The concave side is on the posterior side, so as not to press the normal crystalline lens. The haptics of the lenses that I used were non-vaulted, which assured minimum encroachment on the anterior chamber space and consequently assured maximum possible distance from the corneal endothelium. The thickness of the optic varies from 0.8 to 1.0 mm. The optic size of the early phakic intraocular lens was initially kept at 5 mm and the overall size was 8.5 and even 9 mm. The large size helped to achieve the original concept of Jan Worst of fixing the lens at the peripheral part of the iris (Figs. 19–1 and 19–2). The intraocular lens size was progressively reduced, till after the first 16 cases, the overall size was of the lens was reduced 7.25 mm, whereas the size of the optic diameter was brought near 4.2 mm (Fig. 19–3). We have also used a few convexo-concave lenses, in which the optics at the upper and the lower edges had been cut to give an oval shape to the optic. The optic being convexo-concave in construction, the cutting of the upper and the lower edges, removed the optic edge away from the surface of the iris. Thus in spite of the nonvaulted design, this modification made the optic vaulted in relation to the iris. (Fig. 19–4). The thickest part of the lens, i.e., the center of the optic resides in the deepest part of the anterior chamber. The edges are as thin as 0.17 mm. The thin peripheral thickness of the optic keeps the lens away from the endothelium in the peripheral shallower part of the anterior chamber. This is in contrast to the myopic phakic lenses that have the maximum thickness at the edges of the optics that

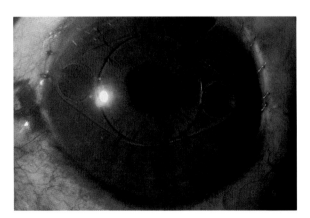

Fig. 19–1. Shows peripheral iris fixation of a plus power lens in a phakic hypermetrope. The claws are symmetrical in this case.

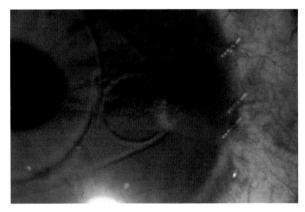

Fig. 19–2. Close up of one of the claws, showing iris inside the claw. There is a linear area of depigmentation, which apparently has been caused by surgical trauma during its passage through the claw.

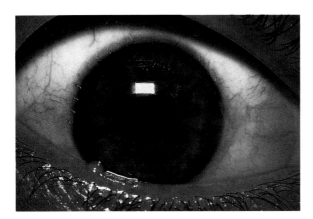

Fig. 19–3. Medium sized convexo-concave iris claw lens. This type of lens has been most used in the present study.

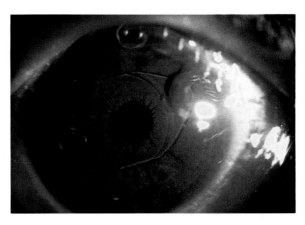

Fig. 19–4. Convexo-concave lens, with the cut upper and the lower edges, that provide a sort of vaulting to the lens.

makes them more prone to the possibility of endothelial touch in case the eye is rubbed. To prevent any intraocular lens contact or pressure on the crystalline lens, the optics of the lenses were made convexo-concave.

Recently, we made a change in the lens design, taking into consideration the peculiar anatomy of the iris. If we look at the normal iris under slit lamp, we usually find that the iris is like a truncated cone. The highest part of the cone appears to be near the area of the collarette, from where there is downward slope towards the pupillary margin (Fig. 19–5). Therefore, it was thought that if the size of the lens could be reduced to a point where the fixation will be near the collarette, then perhaps even convexoplane lens will not put pressure on the crystalline lens. The optic size was therefore reduced to 3.5 mm. It was kept in mind that these cases will need a drop of pilocarpine to avoid edge effect during night time. These 3.5 mm optic mini-lenses can be made thinner than before thereby further increasing the safety to the corneal endothelium. The width of the mini-lenses is 6.5 mm.

The thickness of the haptics is another important matter. It is not known what the ideal thickness of the haptic that will grasp the iris when the pupil is dilated. It seems that the haptic thickness should be around 0.18 mm when the diameter of the claw-ring is 1.2 mm. This is our view when dealing with the brown or black eyes of Indian patients. The claw is fashioned by making a cut in the haptic ring. There is no gap between the two limbs of the claw.

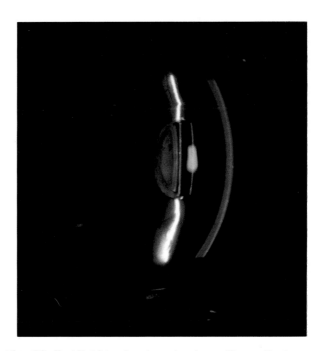

Fig. 19–5. Mini iris-claw lens in place. The optical section shows that the iris is most prominent at the place of the collarette, from where it bends backwards towards the pupil.

Surgical Procedure

All the surgery is done with a head-worn Zeiss 6 X magnification, and illumination is provided from a hand-held source of oblique light. There is no need for a coaxial light operating microscope. The head-worn magnification, gives a freedom of movement to the surgeon's head, so that the surgery is done with the greatest of ease.

The operative techniques have evolved from the earlier to the most recent cases. The earlier method was as follows:

EARLY METHOD

1. A 3 mm two plane limbal incision is made onthe nasal side, just above the 3–9 O'clock line.
2. The pupil is contracted with intracameral carbachol 0.01%.
3. The anterior chamber is filled with hydroxypropylmethylcellulose 2%.
4. A 6 mm two-plane limbal incision is made on the temporal side, just above the 3–9 O'clock line.
5. The anterior chamber is once again deepened with viscoelastic material.
6. The outer small arm of the iris-claw lens is held with a horizontally holding lens for forceps and the lens is slipped inside the anterior chamber. It is firmly held in a centered position. At the same time a special thin iris holding forceps is introduced from the nasal incision. The iris is held and lifted at a suitable place under the long arm of the claw that gets lifted when forward pressure is applied by the forceps. Further forward pressure results in the opening of the claw and the iris preceded by the iris-holding forceps passing through the gap between the two arms of the claw. As soon as the forceps is out of the claw, the claw snaps back and thus grips the iris tissue that has passed through the gap. More iris may be brought into the claw by repeating the process. The quantity of the iris in the claw can be reduced by pushing the iris backwards. Once the fixation of the claw on the nasal side has been achieved, the horizontally

holding as well as the iris holding forceps are withdrawn from the anterior chamber.

7. The anterior chamber is deepened once again with viscoelastic material.
8. The fixation of the temporal claw is done through the larger temporal incision. A vertically holding forceps is used to hold the smaller claw-arm of the temporal haptic. The lens is centered on the pupil and held steady. Now the iris holding forceps is introduced into the anterior chamber, with which the iris tissue is held under the long arm of the temporal claw. Like before, the larger arm of the claw is lifted and the forceps along with the iris is made to pass through the claw. This way, the temporal claw also gets fixed to the iris. Both the lens-holding and the iris-holding forceps are withdrawn. This completes the fixation of the intraocular lens.
9. A peripheral iridectomy is done.
10. Hydroxypropylmethylcellulose is washed out with saline irrigation.
11. The incision line is closed with interrupted 40 micron stainless steel sutures.

SUTURELESS LENS IMPLANTATION

The last 5 cases have been operated in a different manner. Three pocket incisions are made—one being 4.0 mm to 4.5 mm wide at 12 O'clock and the other two being 1 mm wide on the sides. The intraocular lens is slipped into the anterior chamber from the top incision. It is held and centered by a vertically holding forceps, while the tip of only one side of the thin iris forceps is introduced from the side incision. The iris is introduced into the claw by pushing the iris and at the same time lifting the long arm of the claw by the single tip of the iris holding forceps. This extremely simple and effective procedure of iris enclavation was developed by Jenny Rubens of Holland. At the end of the surgery, the corneal dome is lifted with a moderate sized air bubble. After this the anterior chamber is filled with saline so that the eyeball is at a slightly higher than normal intraocular pressure. The air bubble gets absorbed in 3–4 days time. (Figs. 19–6, 19–7, and 19–8).

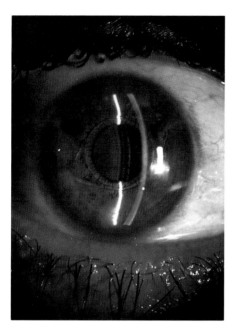

Fig. 19–6. Medium sized convexo-concave iris-claw lens, implanted after making pocket sections and closed without a suture.

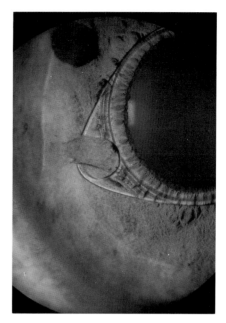

Fig. 19–8. Picture showing the close-up of the claw. The iris is protruding through the claw. An asymmetrical claw has been used in this case, as in most other cases. The shadow of the corneal pocket section is also visible.

PROBLEMS DURING LENS IMPLANTATION

In the early cases, the lack of a viscoelastic material was strongly felt. All the operations in the first year were done under air. Hydroxypropylmethylcellulose 2% when it came to be used by late 1987, was a much better material to work with, however, it has a tendency to flow out during the manipulations in the anterior chamber. The surgery is done usually on relatively young patients, who have elastic eyes. There is tendency for positive pressure from iris-lens side. High hypermetropes frequently have small eyeballs and small corneas. Further the eyes may be so deeply set in the orbit, that all the manipulations for the opening and the closing of the incision line and the acts of lens implantation become extremely difficult.

Immediate Postoperative Problems

There was no postoperative uveitis. Moderate striate keratitis was seen in 6 eyes. Intraocular pressure was raised in 11 eyes, which was treated conservatively.

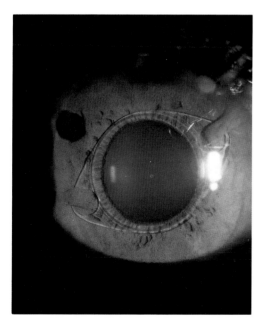

Fig. 19–7. Picture showing the close-up of the convexo-concave iris claw lens in the phakic hypermetropic eye.

Postoperative Medication

Chloramphenical orally for 3 days, prednisolone 20 mg daily for 5 days. Local steroid plus antibiotic drops four times a day for 6 weeks.

RESULTS

The results of the trials are summarized in Table 19–1.

One albino hypermetropic patient received specially made two piece intraocular lenses, the haptics of which were made larger and wider to reduce glare. The patient appreciated the improvement.

One patient with bilateral surgery came for check-up after 52 months. He was found to have chronic iridocyclitis, glaucoma and cataract as well as corneal decompensation in both the eyes. Filteration surgery and explantation were performed in both the eyes. Four months later penetrating keratoplasty was done in one eye, followed by penetrating keratoplasty in the other eye 2 months later. Using aphakic glasses he had visual acuity of 20/40 in the right eye and 20/60 in the left eye. Eleven months later, the grafts showed failure on both sides. Corneal grafting was repeated in the left eye, which again showed signs of failure after 5 months.

Table 19–1. Summary of Clinical Results in 71 Eyes

	Mean	Range	Stnd Dev
Patient Age	26 years	9–52 years	11
Axial length	19.5 mm	15.1–23 mm	1.8 mm
K Values	43.2 D	37–50 diopters	3.5 diopters
AC Depth	3.1 mm	2.3–3.9 mm	0.34 mm
IOL power	15.9 D	9–28 diopters	4.7 D
Follow-up	73.9 mos	3–120 months	29.1 months
Final Refraction (sph equiv)	0.02 D	−5.0 D–3.5 D	2 D
Preop Average Acuity	6/24.8	6/6–6/60	15.7
Postop Average Acuity	6/22.9	6/6–6/60	14

Table 19–2. The Patients Belonged to the Following Age Groups

Age Group	Number
Below 10 Years	2
11–15 Years	12
16–20	8
21–30	28
30–40	12
41–50	8
Over 50 Years	1
Total:	71

Table 19–3. The Axial Length of the Operated Eyes

Axial Length	No.
15–18 mm	12
18+ to 20 mm	28
Over 20 mm	28
Total	68

Table 19–4. K-Readings Varied As Shown Below

Average K (D)	No.
Below 40	18
40+ to 45	34
Over 45	16
Total	68

Table 19–5. The Anterior Chamber Depth

Depth of AC	No.
Below 3 mm	31
3+ to 3.5 mm	26
Over 3.5 mm	5
Total:	62

Table 19–6. The Preoperative Spectacle Power

Spectacle Power	No.
Below +10	46
10+ to 15	17
Over 15 D	5
Total	68

Table 19–7. IOL Powers Used

IOL Power	No.
Below +10	6
10+ to 15	37
15+ to 20	13
20+ to 25	10
Over 25	4
Total:	70

Table 19–8. Follow-Up Period

Period	No.
Below 3 Years	4
3+ to 5 Years	18
5+ to 8 Years	30
8+ to 10 Years	19
Total:	71

Table 19–9. Final Refractive Error

Refraction	No.
−5 to −2 D	6
< −2 to −1	14
< −1 to +1	24
> +1 to +2	17
Over +2	10
Total:	71

Table 19–10. Best Corrected Pre and Postoperative Visual Acuity

BCVA	No. Preop	No. Postop
20/20	2	2
20/30 to 20/40	21	23
20/50 to 20/80	26	26
20/100 to 20/200	22	20
Total:	71	71

Both the corneas showed heavy deep vascularization. Keeping in mind the possibility of failure in further corneal grafts, it was decided to perform keratoprosthesis. A Worst-Singh champagne-cork keratoprosthesis was performed by Dr. Indu R. Singh in the left eye. His corrected vision with −2 sph. recovered to 20/80 with a visual field of 90 + degrees. Earlier, he was a night watchman, but now he is working as a day watchman. The intraocular pressure in both the eyes is well controlled. The vision in the right eye is finger counting at 3 meters. We do not propose to do a keratoprosthesis in this eye as long as the one with a keratoprosthesis is giving good function.

Another patient developed cataract after 18 months. The cause of her cataract is difficult to ascertain. Her intraocular lens was removed and ECCE was done. No intraocular lens was implanted as per her wishes. Her vision with +18 aphakic glass came to 20/80. She is not using any glasses for this eye as the other eye has 20/30 corrected vision.

The endothelial cell counts using specular microscopy were started only recently. The number of the patients studied this far is small so no conclusions can be drawn yet.

DISCUSSION

The first question that arises automatically is, should intraocular lenses be tried in phakic eyes? If we care for the hyperopes, who have a significant visual handicap due to their refractive error, then this trial is not out of place.

Which intraocular lens should be used to manage phakic high hypermetropes? When we started this modality, the only other possible design available was on angle support. The angle support was not chosen because of well-known problems inherent in the angle support system.[1,2]

A pupil support lens was out of question because of the three dimensional nature of the intraocular lens, which was certain to injure the crystalline lens.

Other methods of correction include a soft posterior chamber lens to go between the posterior surface of the iris and the anterior surface of the crystalline lens.[3,4,5] Even if it were available, it was not available at the time would have been thought unsuitable for the purpose, because of the inherent risk of shedding of the posterior iris pigment leading to glaucoma and the risk of interference in the metabolism of the crystalline lens. The formation of adhesions with the iris would also remain a constant possibility.

Our choice fell on iris-support system in the form of an iris-claw lens.[6,7] The word iris-support immediately raises a specter of catastrophe, that is commonly associated with the earlier used pupillary lenses. These lenses had two great drawbacks—dislocation and corneal decompensation. The dislocation occurred because the three-dimensional construction of the lens was loosely supported by the pupil. As soon as the pupil dilated, the lens would fall into the anterior chamber. It had to be replaced or explanted. The corneal decompensation was due to a variety of factors. The major cause was, to my mind, the use of an unphysiological miotic (Miochol) that in those days was formulated in distilled water. It is only after 1986 that saline has been used instead of distilled water. By this time the pupil supported or iris sutured lenses had disappeared in the United States. The other contributory factors to corneal decompensation were relatively inexperienced implant surgeons and their less than sophisticated tools, lack of understanding about corneal endothelium or the facilities for specular

endothelial microscopy, and the nonavailability of viscoelastic agents.

I was fortunate, practicing in India, not to suffer from the unphysiological-miotic induced corneal decompensation. I made my own intraocular miotic in lactated Ringer solution. Many of my earliest patients with pupil supported lenses implanted after ICCE are still alive with healthy corneas and good endothelial cell counts, nearly 19 years after surgery. My switch over from pupil-supported to the iris supported (iris-claw lens) was smooth, since it removed the major objection of the former design, the dislocation. We did face surgical and postsurgical problems due to the nonavailability of a cost effective viscoelastic material. The availability of hydroxypropylmethylcellulose (HPMC) 2% in 1988 gave us a sigh of relief. Whereas in the United States, the pupil-support (miscalled iris-fixation) disappeared, we in India became more confident in the form of an iris-claw lens in the aphakic eye and later in the phakic eye.

The iris-claw lens implantation for phakic hypermetropes was selected on the presumption that the other available methods for treating high hypermetropia, appeared far less promising. Our extensive and intensive experience with iris-claw lenses gave us the assurance about the short and the long term safety of the procedure. The possibility of atraumatic explantation in case it was needed, was also available. Unfortunately one patient due to lack of availability of correct and timely aid, suffered severe complications.

In today's context, an intraocular lens in a phakic hypermetrope has a place, because the surgery is straight forward and relatively atraumatic. The results are predictable and immediate. As compared to minus lenses for phakic myopes, the hyperopia lens appears safer. The reason is that although the myopia lens is thickest at the edges, the hyperopia lens is thinnest at the edges. The result is that there are lesser chances of endothelial touch.

Drawbacks of Intraocular Lenses in the Phakic Eye

The patient should not rub the eye. This is a life long precaution. The eye should be examined periodically. A regular follow-up is necessary, with a special care to the counting of the endothelial cells. Later in

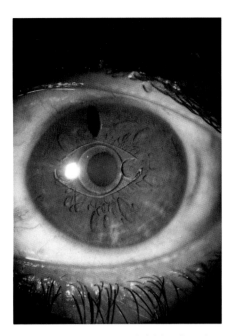

Fig. 19–9. Picture showing mini iris-claw lens of convexo-plane construction, fixed to the most prominent part of the iris cone at the collarette.

life, when a patient develops cataract, it should be possible for any surgeon to explant this lens under cover of a viscoelastic material.

Recently mini plano-convex lenses have been used. They have an optic of 3.5 mm and an overall width of 6.8 mm (Fig. 19–9). The idea behind the use of mini-plano-convex lenses is as follows. The iris is in the form of a truncated cone. The highest part of the iris coincides with the collarette. From collarette towards the pupillary margin, the iris bends backwards. Therefore, if a lens is fixed at the collarette, it will remain clear of the crystalline lens. If a drop of pilocarpine is instilled, it will reduce the possibility of touching the crystalline and it will also avoid the edge-effect at night time. There may be a little difficulty at night time due to a small pupil, but it is a small price to pay for the benefits of a mini-plano-convex lens. The idea has appeared to work in the few cases that have been done. However, ours is

not an automobile driving society. It is my perception that I felt more comfortable and at peace with convexo-concave lenses than the latest mini-plano-convex lenses.

CONCLUSIONS

Lens implantation in the phakic hyperopic eyes deserves further study. There is no better teacher than a failure, which shows us newer directions for research. However, if any research in this field has to be meaningful, it should be free from prejudice and dogma. At the same time, we should look towards the coming results of more easily applicable and less invasive techniques like PRK and LASIK.

REFERENCES

1. Leroux les Jardins S, Heligon JP, Ozdemir N, et al: Medium-term tolerance of anterior chamber implants in surgical treatment of severe myopia. *J Fr Ophtalmol* 18(1):45–49, 1995.
2. Kashani AA: Fluorophotometry in myopic phakic eyes with anterior chamber intraocular lenses to correct severe myopia (letter, comment). *Am J Ophthalmol* 119(3):381–382, 1995.
3. Fechner PU, Haigis W, Wichmann W: Posterior chamber myopia lenses in phakic eyes. *J Cataract Refract Surg* 2:178–182, 1996.
4. Erturk H, Ozcetin H: Phakic posterior chamber intraocular lenses for the correction of high myopia. *J Refract Surg* 11(5):388–391, 1995.
5. Ibrahim O, Waring G: Successful exchange of dislocated phakic intraocular lens. *J Refract Surg* 11(4):282–283, 1995.
6. Landesz M, Worst JG, Siertsema JV, van Rij G: Correction of high myopia with the Worst myopia claw intraocular lens. *J Refract Surg* 11(1):16–25, 1995.
7. Menezo JL, Cisneros A, Hueso JR, Harto M: Long-term results of surgical treatment of high myopia with Worst-Fechner intraocular lenses. *J Cataract Refract Surg* 21(1):93–98, 1995.

section VII
Other Modalities

CHAPTER 20

Small Diameter Intracorneal Inlay Lens for the Correction of Presbyopia

Richard L. Lindstrom

INTRODUCTION

Large diameter intracorneal lenses have been utilized in the past for the correction of refractive errors such as myopia (nearsightedness) and hyperopia (farsightedness).[1-5] This chapter discusses the development of an intracorneal lens that is a small diameter hydrogel corneal lens (SDICL) for the correction of presbyopia. The purpose of the lens is to reduce the patient's dependence on reading glasses or bifocals.

Treatment for presbyopia has traditionally involved the use of reading glasses, bifocal spectacles or bifocal contact lenses. The power of a lens is measured in diopters and the add power required to correct presbyopia ranges from +1.00 to +4.00 diopters to allow clear focus on an object held at a comfortable reading distance. In a bifocal eyeglass, the individual chooses either to look through the distance portion or the near portion depending on the location of the object to be viewed.

Some recent contact lens and intraocular lens designs rely on a concept called simultaneous vision where the near and distance focusing elements are within the optical zone of the eye at the same time.[6,7] The brain preferentially selects the near or distant object without having to move the eye to look through the distance or near portion of the lens. The brain essentially selects the more focused image on the retina over the unfocused image without confusion.

The small diameter intracorneal inlay lens design uses the normal human cornea as one of the major focusing lenses of the eye measuring approximately 43.50 diopters.

The central optical power of the normal human cornea is fairly uniform over the central optical zone resulting in a single focus plane on the retina. In order to correct presbyopia with the small diameter intracorneal inlay lens a 2 mm diameter +2.00 to +4.00 diopter powered lens is placed in the central area of the cornea to create a bifocal cornea. When the small diameter intracorneal inlay lens is implanted into the optic zone of the cornea (Fig. 20–1) it produces a region in the center of the cornea that has a higher refractive power due to the lens design and power.

Light from a distant object passes through the unmodified portion of the cornea and is focused on the retina allowing a clear view of distant objects. Another portion of the light passing through the cornea, passes through the inlay and is focused anterior to the retina when viewing a distant object. Creating an unfocused image that is basically ignored by the brain (Fig. 20–2A). Conversely, when viewing a near object, the light from the near object passes through the inlay portion of the cornea and is focused directly on the retina resulting in a clear image of the near object whereas the light passing through the unmodified portion of the cornea is defocused posterior to the retina and is again ignored by the brain (Fig. 20–2B).

Clinical trials with multifocal contact lenses and intraocular lenses have demonstrated that the human visual system is able to select the in focus image so that both near and distant objects can be seen clearly, alternately, at the discretion of the individual. The small diameter intracorneal inlay lens is based on the same optical principle.

CURRENT SURGICAL TECHNIQUE

The surgical procedure takes approximately 15 minutes in an outpatient surgical setting and can be performed under topical anesthesia.

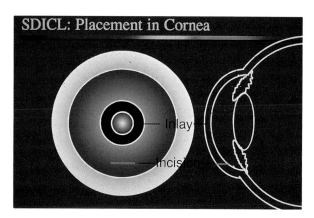

Fig. 20–1. Schematic of placement of hydrogel inlay in cornea. A 2.5 mm long incision is made parallel and approximately 1 mm from the limbus with a diamond knife. This incision is set at approximately 75% of corneal thickness.

A 2.5 mm long incision is made parallel and approximately 1 mm from the limbus with a diamond knife. This incision is set at approximately 75% of corneal thickness based on measurement of the corneal thickness by pachymetry.

The knives utilized are similar to the knives utilized in radial and astigmatic keratotomy.[8,9] The incision can be made on the steeper meridian of the cornea resulting in reduction of the patient's astig-

matism. A small spatula is utilized to dissect a pocket to the center of the cornea. The small diameter intracorneal inlay lens is then placed on the spatula and centered over the patient's pupil. No sutures are required as the incision is self healing. Intraoperative and postoperative discomfort is minimal. No patch is required. Visual recovery is rapid. Postoperative care includes the use of a topical antibiotic and a steroid combination drop for 1 to 4 weeks.

LENS DESIGN

The lenses under study range from 1.8 to 2.2 mm in diameter and are made from a hydrogel polymer with a water content of 45%. This is basically the same material utilized in a soft contact lens (Fig. 20–3). The flexibility of this material enables the lens to easily conform to the shape of the cornea and minimizes any scarring and remodeling. Hydrogel has a refractive index of 1.425 as compared to the normal corneal refractive index of 1.376 that allows an effective power of the lens in the range of +1 to +4 diopters with a very thin implant. The lens thickness in this power range is only 30 to 60 microns whereas the normal central corneal thickness is approximately 530 microns.

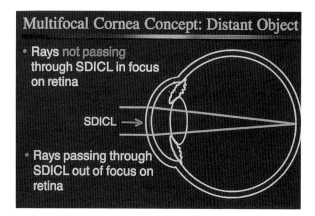

Fig. 20–2A. Multifocal concept of intracorneal lenses for distant objects. Rays not passing through intracorneal lenses (SDICL) will be in focus on retina and rays passing through the intracorneal lens will not be in focus.

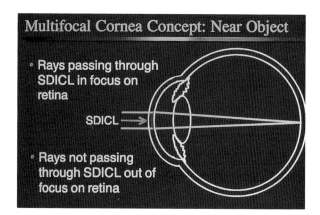

Fig. 20–2B. Multifocal cornea concept for Near. Rays passing through the intracorneal lens (SDICL) will be in focus on the retina and rays not passing through the intracorneal lens will be out of focus on retina.

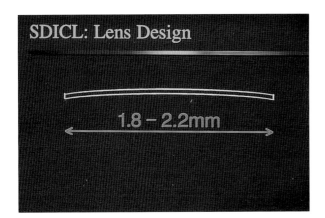

Fig. 20–3. Schematic of small diameter intracorneal lens.

Since the anterior cornea receives its nutrients from the aqueous media, the lens needs to be permeable to glucose and other nutrient materials. Hydrogel material allows transport of glucose through its stroma due to its high water content.[10] Hydrogel inlays have been safely implanted into the cornea of primates[11,12,13] and humans[14] for extended periods and have been shown to be safe. Unlike a contact lens on the surface of the eye, the small diameter intracorneal lens does not interfere with oxygen transport to the cornea, especially the metabolically active epithelial layer. This may well make it better tolerated than many contact lenses.

EXPERIMENTAL STUDIES IN ANIMALS

Inlays implanted in rabbits and cats were found to be well tolerated. The material was shown to be inert and nonirritative. In addition, the procedure was shown to be reversible in animal studies that means that a patient who is not satisfied with the result can have the intraocular lens removed or exchanged.

Table 20–1. Design Specifications

- Meniscus lens
- 45% Hydrogel: Helflcon-A
- Thickness: 0.03 to 0.06 mm
- Diameter: 1.80 to 2.20 mm
- Resolution: ≥ 3/4 AFTR

HUMAN CLINICAL TRIALS

Initially, the lenses were implanted into nonsighted eyes in Australia and South America. Small diameter intracorneal inlay lenses remained clear and deposit free as expected. The surgical pockets quickly retained clarity and were difficult to see as early as one week after surgery. Two months after implantation reversibility was demonstrated by removal of inlays with return of the cornea to its normal configuration. Evaluation of the corneal surface curvature showed no significant induced astigmatism or spherical refractive error.

In 1994, Chiron Vision opened an investigational device exemption (IDE) under the auspices of the United States Food and Drug Administration.

Three United States surgeon investigators were selected as well as one Australian and one South American Ophthalmologist. To date, 23 patients have received small diameter intracorneal inlay lenses for presbyopia ranging in diameter from 1.8 to 2.2 mm and in power from +2.20 to +3.5 diopters. Richard L. Lindstrom, M.D., at the Phillips Eye Institute in Minneapolis has implanted 11 lenses, Daniel S. Durrie, M.D. of Kansas City has implanted 6, Graham Barrett, M.D. (the inlay inventor) of Perth, Australia has implanted 4, Richard Keates, M.D. of Irvine, California and Roberto Zaldivar, M.D. of Buenos Aires, Argentina have each implanted 1. The first implants were placed in June of 1994 and are just now achieving their one year postoperative follow-up inside the international multicenter trial. The results in general reveal that all patients achieve improved uncorrected near acuity. Results are shown below for 23 eyes with 1 to 9 months follow-up. Table 20–2 shows pre and postoperative visions.

Patients with the more powerful 3.5 diopter intracorneal lens have all achieved an equivalent of 20/20

Table 20–2. Small Diameter Intracorneal Inlay Lens for Presbyopia Clinical Results: All Cases

1–9 months follow-up	>20/20	20/25 20/40	20/50 20/100	20/200 or worse
Preop UCVA			15	8
Postop UCVA	7	4	7	5

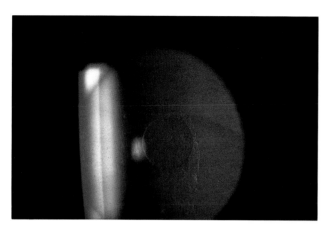

Fig. 20–4A. Red Reflex Photo of Postoperative Intracorneal Lens

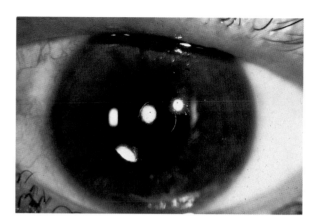

Fig. 20–4B. Different view of same eye without dilation.

vision at near without correction by six months after surgery. Patients with the less powerful 2.0 to 2.5 diopter adds have achieved near visions ranging from 20/20 to 20/100. Figures 20–4A and B show an eye with a small diameter intracorneal lens months after surgery.

Table 20–3 below shows the best and worst case examples and the uncorrected and best corrected near and distance vision.

Table 20–4 shows the breakdown of which power implants were used.

COMPLICATIONS

Most patients have noticed a small decrease in the quality of their best corrected vision at distance which has varied from a few letters to a full line on a Snellen visual acuity chart. Two of the 23 patients have been unsatisfied and requested that the lens be removed. In both these cases, the cornea and visual status of the patient returned to its preoperative levels with no loss of acuity or visual function. There were no cases of inflammation, infection, corneal opacity, irritation or melt.

Thirty-nine percent of patients lost 2 lines or more of uncorrected distance acuity and 30.4% lost two lines or more of best corrected distance acuity. No patients lost 2 or more lines of uncorrected or best corrected near vision. *See* Table 20–5.

The preliminary results with the small diameter intracorneal inlay lens for presbyopia are promising. An additional group of patients is expected to be implanted with a slightly larger 2.2 mm version with an effective power of approximately +3.00 to +3.50 diopters in the near future. Once the ideal

Table 20–3. Best Case/Worst Case Examples

		UCVA Distance	Near	BCVA Distance	Near
Presbyope	pre	20/30	20/60	20/16	20/20
3.5D SDICL	post	20/20	20/20	20/16	20/20
Pseudophake	pre	20/30	20/100	20/20	20/20
3.5D SDICL	post	20/30	20/20	20/25	20/20
Pseudophake	pre	20/30	20/50	20/25	20/20
3.5D SDICL	post	20/40	20/200	20/25	20/25
(removed)					

Table 20–4. Clinical Results All Cases

N = 23, 1–9 mos follow-up
3.5 D: (5) removed 0
2.5 D: (13) removed 1, inadequate near
2.0 D (5) removed 1, inadequate near

Table 20–5. Adverse Reactions/Complications[a]

Loss of ≥ 2 Lines UC Distance	(9)	39.1%
Loss of ≥ 2 Lines UC Near	(0)	0
Loss of ≥ 2 Lines BC Distance	(7)	30.4%
Loss of ≥ 2 Lines BC Near	(0)	0

[a]n = 23; 1–9 months follow-up, UC, uncorrected, BC, best corrected

size and power parameters are determined the study will be expanded to a multicenter investigation of several hundred patients in pursuit of pre-market approval in the United States. In addition, parallel investigations will continue in Australia, South America and Europe.

SUMMARY

Presbyopia is a condition that affects humans over the age of 45 resulting in the need to utilize reading glasses or bifocals for near work. The etiology of this condition is a loss of the ability of the normal lens of the eye to accommodate or focus on near objects. A novel device and surgical procedure has been developed for the correction of this condition. A small lens, approximately 2 mm in diameter and +2.00 to +4.00 diopters in power is implanted into the optical zone of the human cornea at approximately 75% depth. This produces a multifocal cornea capable of focusing both near and distance objects onto the retina. The visual system works similar to the visual system in a bifocal contact lens or intraocular lens. The brain is able to sort out the images cast on the retina, providing either a clear near or distance image. The intracorneal inlay lens is produced by from a hydrogel copolymer with a water content of 45% and a refractive index of

1.425. The lenses are currently being implanted in the United States, Australia, and Argentina by five surgeons under an investigational device exemption from the United States Food and Drug Administration. They are manufactured by Chiron Vision of Claremont, California.

REFERENCES

1. McCarey BE: Refractive keratoplasty with synthetic lens implants. *Int Ophthalmol Clin* 31:87, 1991.
2. Lindstrom RL, Lane SS: Polysulfone intracorneal lenses. In DR Saunders, RF Hoffman, JJ Salz: *Refractive Corneal Surgery.* New Jersey, Slack, 1986, pp 551–563.
3. McCarey BE: Alloplastic refractive keratoplasty; Ibid. pp 531–548.
4. Maxwell WA, Nordan LT: *Current Concepts of Multifocal Intraocular Lenses.* New Jersey, Slack, 1991.
5. Barrett GD, Link WJ, Reich CJ: Refractive Bifocal Corneal Inlay Lenses. U.S. Patent No. 5.196.026.
6. Ravalico G, Baccara F, Bellavitis A: Refractive bifocal intraocular lens and pupillary diameters. *J Cataract Refract Surg* 18:594, 1992.
7. Ravalico G, Baccara F, Bellavitis A: Contrast sensitivity in multifocal intraocular lenses. *J Cataract Refract Surg* 19:22, 1993.
8. Waring III GO ed: *Refractive Keratotomy for Myopia and Astigmatism.* Missouri, Mosby-Year Book, Inc., 1992.
9. Binder PS, Waring III GO: Keratotomy for astigmatism, pp 1085–1198.
10. McCarey BE, Schmidt FH: Modeling glucose distribution in the cornea. *Current Eye Research,* 9:1025, 1990.
11. McCarey BE, McDonald MB, van Rij G, et al: Refractive results of hyperopic hydrogel intracorneal lenses in primate eyes. *Arch Ophthalmol* 107:724, 1989.
12. McCarey BE, van Rij G: Refractive predictability of myopic hydrogel intracorneal lenses in primate eyes. *Arch Ophthalmol* 108:1310, 1990.
13. Werblin TP, Peiffer RL, Binder PS, McCarey BE, Patel AS: Eight years experience with Permalens intracorneal lenses in nonhuman primates. *Refract Corneal Surg* 8:12, 1992.
14. Werblin TP, Patel AS, Barraquer JI: Initial human experience with Permalens myopic hydrogel intracorneal lens implants. *Refract Corneal Surg* 8:23, 1992.

CHAPTER 21

The Corneal Contouring Device for Hyperopia

Richard A. Eiferman
Robert Nordquist, Ph.D.

INTRODUCTION

A simple mechanical device to correct farsightedness was conceived and designed by the late Gene Reynolds, O.D., M.D., Ph.D. Dr. Reynolds theorized that, if the central or peripheral cornea could be reproducibly steepened or flattened, then the surgical correction of refractive errors was possible.

Many years ago, he recognized that the diameter of concentric rings projected onto the cornea was mathematically related to the dioptric power of the cornea at each ring. This principle was embodied in his classic invention, the corneascope, as well as in his models of the corneal comparator.[1,2,3] Using his knowledge of corneal topography, he devised a new nomogram that calculated the amount of peripheral flattening that would be necessary to reshape the cornea for the correction of hyperopia.

Historical Review of the Current Technique

Dr. Reynolds designed a simple mechanical device for selective removal of corneal tissue. The corneal contouring device (CCD) consists of a double vacuum chamber constructed of Lucite (Fig. 21–1). The outer ring is applied to the limbus that attaches the CCD to the eye and provides centration; the inner ring has a 8.0 mm diameter and draws a higher vacuum (Fig. 21–2). Steel blades are mounted orthogonally on a central piston that can be lowered by a micrometer into the inner chamber. As the pressure is elevated, the cornea is flattened within the chamber and can be predictably cut by the rotating blades.

The Theory of CCD

The corneal contouring device utilizes the principle of lamellar corneal dissection. Early experiments indicated that it was very difficult to mechanically cut a spherical surface, but the process was greatly simplified when it is planar. When corneal fibers are put on stretch, the rotating blades progressively delaminate the collagen fibrils analogous to a carpenter's plane.

Early studies in human bank eyes revealed that high speeds of rotation had very little effect as the blades tended to hydroplane over the surface. However, much slower speeds (in the range of 30 to 60 oscillations per minute), allowed the blades to consecutively peel the collagen lamellae. Progressive horizontal cuts were ineffective, but an oscillating blade mounted orthogonally with small honing angles consistently produced long strips of collagen. Furthermore, each sweep progressively smoothed and polished the previous pass.

Surgery for correction of hyperopia requires a large optical zone. This is very difficult to achieve with the excimer laser: doubling the area of the ablation zone requires squaring the power of the laser. A mechanical device can easily achieve a large optical zone by increasing the diameter of the inner tube; removal of more tissue from the periphery than the center creates a hyperopic lens. This can be achieved by placing a 3 mm teflon button in the center of the piston (Fig. 21–3). This protects and prevents any cutting of the central cornea while simultaneously causing the periphery to bulge against the walls of the chamber. As the blade is progressively lowered, only peripheral tissue is removed which

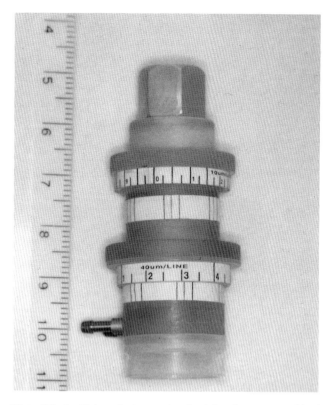

Fig. 21-1. This photograph depicts the assembled Corneal Contouring device with the blade in place. Note that the total length of the device is only 6 cm.

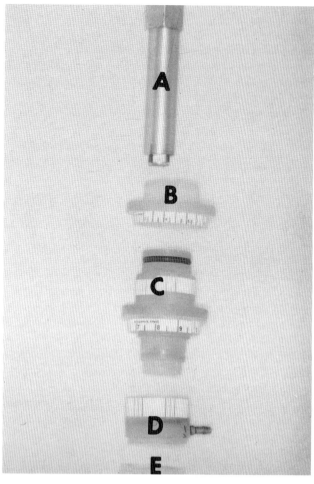

Fig. 21-2. This Figure is an exploded view of the C.C.D. device showing (a) the knife, (b) the micrometer dial for depth of cut, (c) the body of the device that rests against the cornea with its bottom surface, (d) the vacuum manifold and scleral ring mount, and (e) the scleral ring.

effectively steepens the central cornea. Approximately four diopters of hyperopic correction can be achieved with this technique.

SURGICAL TECHNIQUE

Under topical anesthesia, the instrument is attached to the limbus by engaging the vacuum ring. When adequate fixation is achieved, the inner chamber vacuum is applied. The cutting blades are lowered until the epithelium is encountered. They are then further lowered under micrometer control to the desired setting (which is derived from the nomogram). The blades are rotated; the initial passes remove the epithelium in the periphery and then into stroma. A circular cut can be seen spreading centripetally that stops at the central post. At that time, no additional tissue can be removed; further rotations of the piston serve to "polish" the bed.

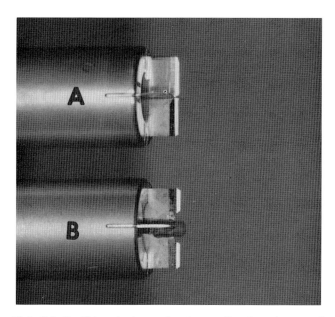

Fig. 21–3. This photograph shows the two types of blades used in the C.D.D. device. Blade A is the blade to achieve a myopic cut. Blade B is the hyperopic cut. Note the central button and gaps in the blades centrally.

Animal Studies of Wound Healing

The CCD procedure was performed on cats and owl monkeys. Many animals developed a post operative perilimbal subconjunctival hemorrhage from the suction ring that resolved spontaneously. Epithelialization was usually complete at three days. Periodic slit lamp examination revealed no evidence of subepithelial haze. The corneas remained clear and the anterior chamber and crystalline lens were unaffected.

Histopathology

Light and electron microscopic studies performed immediately following the procedure revealed the paracentral epithelium was easily removed by the rotating blades, but the central 3 mm was spared (Fig. 21–4). As Bowman's layer and the stroma is encountered, an exceptionally uniform transitional zone is created using this technique (Figs. 21–5 to 21–12). It should be noted the edge is feathered for 360° which flows smoothly into the underlying stromal bed. This is minimal damage to the collagen

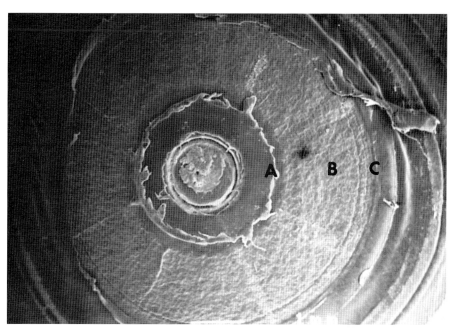

Fig. 21–4. Scanning electron micrograph of a hyperopic cut on a cat cornea. This specimen was not washed or cleaned after the operation in order to observe the residual debris. Note the central island. Though the epithelium is marred in a circular manner in the center, the 3.5 mm diameter central island was spared. The following three scanning electron micrographs will show the detail of the areas labeled A, B, and C in this picture.(×18)

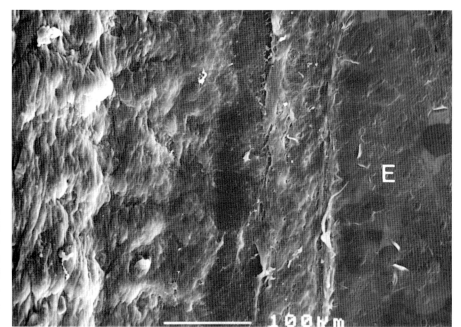

Fig. 21–5. The position in this photograph is shown in Fig. 21–4 labeled A. This SEM is a high magnification of the area of transition from the edge of the central island to the deep stroma. The epithelium (E) is undamaged and contains light and dark cells.(×300)

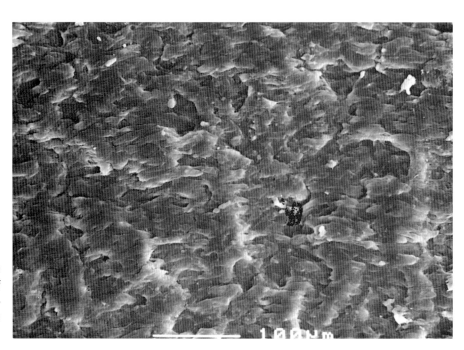

Fig. 21–6. This SEM shows the collagen surface in the center of the hyperopic cut. This photograph was taken in the position marked B on Fig. 4.(×300)

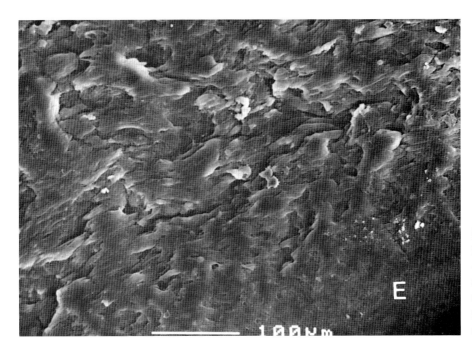

Fig. 21–7. This picture was taken from the position marked C in Fig. 4. This photograph shows the transition from the outside epithelium outside the hyperopic cut and its transition to the stroma. The epithelium is labeled E.(×700)

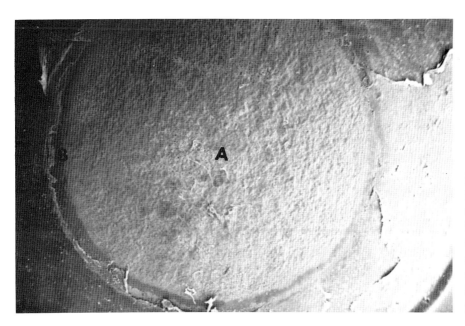

Fig. 21–8. This SEM shows a myopic cut with an 8 mm optical zone. Note the smooth surface of the cut. This specimen was not washed or cleaned in order to observe the residual debris. High magnification of detail of the sites labeled A and B will be seen in the next two photographs.(×22)

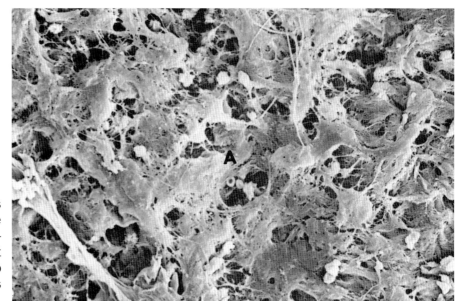

Fig. 21–9. This photograph shows a high magnification SEM of the central ablation zone of the specimen shown in Fig. 21–8. Note that this cut has entered the deep stroma as evidenced by the gaps in the collagen lamella.(×750)

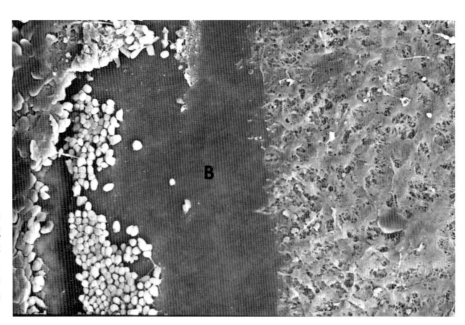

Fig. 21–10. This photograph is a high magnification SEM showing the feathered edge of the cut that begins at the epithelium (E), feathers smoothly into Bowman's membrane (B), then descends into the stroma (S).(×300)

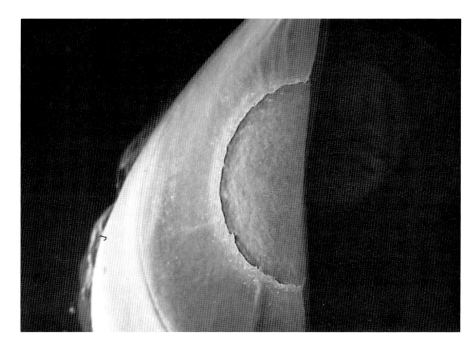

Figure 21.11. This SEM depicts a myopic cut in a cat cornea which has been bisected for further study.(×18)

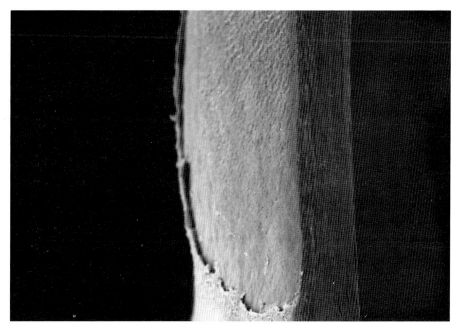

Fig. 21–12. This photograph is a high magnification SEM to show the cut edge of the central cornea immediately after the C.C.D. procedure.(×75)

lamellae and a negligible inflammatory response. The endothelium and Descemet's membrane are unaffected.

Long-term healing studies in primates undergoing CCD surgery were almost indistinguishable from the excimer laser after two years.[4-11] However, none of the animals developed subepithelial "haze" or recurrent erosions. Bowman's layer was absent centrally with minimal duplication of the basal lamina (Figs. 21–13 to 21–15) and the subadjacent tissue is unaffected.

While the healing patterns were very similar to the excimer laser, animals often demonstrated marked reduplication of the basal lamina after PRK. The deep stroma, descemet's membrane and endothelium remained normal.

Corneal Topography

Owl monkeys have a central corneal curvature similar to humans. Preliminary studies indicate up to three diopters of corneal steepening can be consistently achieved which remain stable for at least two years.

CONCLUSION

The corneal contouring device is a promising instrument for hyperopic surgery. Long-term human trials are planned.

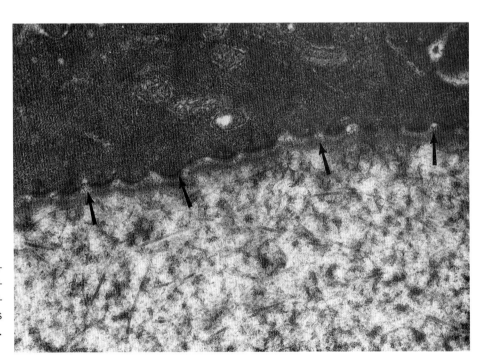

Fig. 21–13. This is a transmission electron micrograph showing the basal lamina of a normal primate cornea. Arrows indicate the basal lamina. (×20,000)

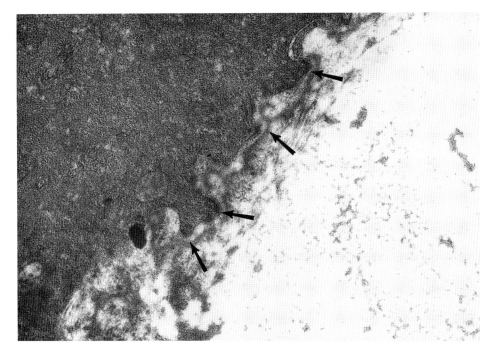

Fig. 21–14. This photograph is a TEM of a primate cornea two years following the C.C.D. procedure. At surgery this eye was projected for a 3 diopter cut. At the end of two years post-op, the eye had a 2.5 diopter correction. This photograph shows the basal lamina (arrows). it can be noted that although there are some oblique cuts, there is very little, if any, duplication of the basal lamina.(×20,000)

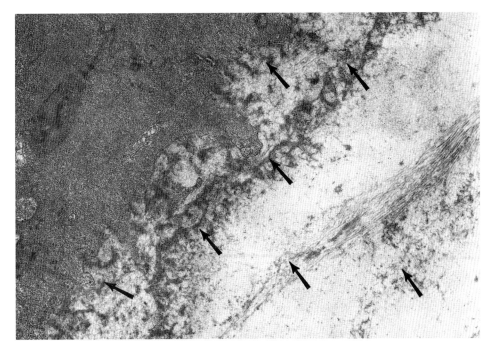

Fig. 21–15. This photograph is a TEM of a primate cornea two years after PRK with a Taunton LV2000 excimer laser. This animal was treated to produce a 6 diopter myopic correction. At two years post-op, there was only 3 diopters remaining. The arrows indicate the basal lamina and its many duplications. This generally indicates the epithelium has been removed and replaced many times. (×20,000)

REFERENCES

1. Rowsey JJ: Ten caveats in keratorefractive surgery. *Ophthalmology* 90:148–155, 1983.
2. Waring GO: *Refractive Keratotomy for Myopia and Astigmatism.* St. Louis, Mosby-Year Book, 1992.
3. Doss JD, Hutson RL, Rowsey JJ, Brown OR: Method for the calculation of corneal profile and power distribution. *Arch Ophthalmol* 99:1261–1265, 1981.
4. Gaster, McCord R, Berns MW, Burstein NL: Excimer laser ablation and wound healing of superficial cornea in rabbits and primates. *Invest Ophthalmol Vis Sci* 29:309, 1988.
5. Kerr-Muir MG, Trokel SL, Marshall J, Rothery S: Ultrastructural comparison of conventional surgical and argon fluoride excimer laser keratectomy. *Am J Ophthalmol* 103:448, 1987.
6. McDonald M, Frantz J, Santana E, Salmeron B, Klyce S, Beverman R, Kaufman H: Excimer laser surface shaping of the primate cornea for the correction of myopia. *Invest Ophthalmol Vis Sci* 29:310, 1988.
7. McDonald MB, Frantz JM, Klyce SD, Beverman RW, Varnell R, Munnerlyn CR, Clapham TN, Salmeron B, Kaufman HE: Central photorefractive keratectomy for myopia: The blind eye study. *Arch Ophthalmol* 108:799, 1990.
8. Fantes FE, Hanna KD, Waring GO, Pouliquen Y, Thompson KP, Savoldelli M: Wound healing after excimer laser keratomileusis (photorefractive keratectomy) in monkeys. *Arch Ophthalmol* 108:665, 1990.
9. Hanna v, Pouliquen YM, Savoldelli M, Fantes F, Thompson KP, Waring III GO, Samson J: Corneal wound healing in monkeys 18 months after excimer laser photorefractive keratectomy. *Refract Corneal Surg* 6:340, 1990.
10. Malley DS, Steinert RF, Puliafito CA, Dob ET: Immunofluorescence study of corneal wound healing after excimer laser anterior keratectomy in the monkey eye. *Arch Ophthalmol* 108:1316–1322, 1990.
11. Tuft SJ, Zabel RW, Marshall J: Corneal repair following keratectomy: A comparison between conventional surgery and laser photoablation. *Invest Ophthalmol Vis Sci* 30:1769–1777, 1989.

Index

Page numbers in italic indicate figures. Page numbers followed by "t" indicate tables.

211